I0786984

The Early Years of the Chronic Fatigue Syndrome Epidemic Cover-up

1981-1989

Charles Ortleb

Published by HHV-6 University Press, Salem, Massachusetts

PRINTED IN THE UNITED STATES OF AMERICA

ISBN: 9798709847446

10 9 8 7 6 5 4 3 2 1
First Edition

A Note from the Publisher

This volume contains the first six chapters from *The Chronic Fatigue Syndrome Epidemic Cover-up: How a Little Newspaper Solved the Biggest Scientific and Political Mystery of Our Time.*

From 1980-1997, a little newspaper in New York found itself at the center of one of the darkest chapters in the history of science and medicine. In *Rolling Stone*, David Black said *New York Native* deserved a Pulitzer Prize for its pioneering reporting on the AIDS epidemic. The number of important stories *New York Native* broke about AIDS, Chronic Fatigue Syndrome, and AIDS fraud should have guaranteed several Pulitzer Prizes. Even Randy Shilts acknowledged the *New York Native*'s unique coverage of AIDS in *And the Band Played On.* But the uncompromising nature of *New York Native*'s investigative reporting ultimately made it a thorn in the establishment's side. The moral of the *New York Native* story is that no important and independent journalism goes unpunished. Books by Larry Kramer, David France, and others have disparaged and distorted the history and legacy of *New York Native*. It's time to correct the record.

In 1989, Katie Leishman wrote in *Rolling Stone*, "It is undeniable that many major stories were Ortleb's months and sometimes years before mainstream journalism took them up."

For Francis and everyone who worked at
or supported the *New York Native*.

Contents

Introduction 11

1981-1984: The Fog of Epidemiology 15

1985: Throwing Down the Gauntlet 40

1986: A New Virus or a Renamed Old One? 82

1987: An Epic Epidemiological Battle 110

1988: The Public Relations of the Epidemic 137

1989: A Strategy Emerges...162

Notes 191

Introduction

The history of epidemics, narrowly studied, does not suggest
the risks of the great plague to come that will dominate the
planet.
—Nassim Nicholas Taleb, *The Black Swan*

In *The March of Folly*, Barbara Tuchman uses the word "folly" to
describe periods in history of egregious, self-defeating misgovernment, and one of her most dramatic examples of folly is America's
catastrophic policies during the Vietnam era. I think that the AIDS and
"chronic fatigue syndrome (CFS)" era would have easily fulfilled the
requirements of her definition of folly or counterproductive
misgovernment, and in terms of the medical and social damage that
the foolishness of the AIDS/CFS era has caused and is still causing,
Vietnam by comparison starts to look like a minor example of the
political vice she describes.

Tuchman identifies periods of government folly as ones in which
policies are pursued which run counter to a government's best
interests. They are periods of presumptuousness and hubris that
practically beg the gods for comeuppance. They are the times in history
that prompt one to ask, "What were they thinking?" They involve
"woodenheadedness" and massive "self-deception." Governments,
frozen in "fixed belief," ignore all "evidence to the contrary" that
warns them away from the precipice of disaster. Essentially, during
Tuchmanesque periods of "folly," governments stop thinking and
forsake common sense and sound judgment.

To qualify for Tuchman's certificate of "folly," a "policy adapted
must meet three criteria: it must have been perceived as counterproductive in its own time, not merely by hindsight." The second
criterion is, "a feasible alternative course of action must have been
available." And the third criterion is, "that the policy should be that of
a group, not an individual ruler."

For any jury of historians that tries to determine if the AIDS era
truly satisfies Tuchman's criteria for a judgment of folly, I offer *New
York Native* as Exhibit A for the prosecution. During the formative
years of the AIDS epidemic the critical reporting and editorials of the
New York Native continually pointed out that the AIDS/CFS policies
of the government and the AIDS establishment were "wooden-

headed" and counterproductive. As the folly of the epidemic proceeded inexorably, *New York Native* made it abundantly clear that there was a feasible alternative to the catastrophically mistaken, bigoted politics, epidemiology and virology of AIDS and "chronic fatigue syndrome" that concealed one shocking multisystemic pandemic. And as the horrific story of the epidemic unfolded in relentless detail in the pages of *New York Native*, it became painfully obvious that there was plenty of blame to pass around and no single individual was the unifying tyrant completely controlling this dystopian period of biomedical totalitarianism and abnormal science. The demise of *New York Native,* which itself came under fire from the gay community (as well as the AIDS and "chronic fatigue syndrome" establishment) for its diligent and inconvenient truth-telling, is just another layer of the epidemic's tragic folly.

*

Ron Rosenbaum devotes a chapter of his fascinating book, *Explaining Hitler: The Search for the Origins of His Evil,* to the *Munich Post,* the fearless newspaper which Hitler's party referred to as "the Poison Kitchen." According to Rosenbaum, the newspaper was Hitler's "nemesis," "the persistent poisoned thorn in his side." Rosenbaum wrote, "The *Munich Post* journalists were the first to focus sustained critical attention on Hitler, from the very first moments this strange specter emerged from the beer-hall backrooms to take to the streets of Munich in the early 1920s. They were the first to tangle with him, the first to ridicule him, the first to investigate him, the first to expose the seamy underside of his party, the murderous criminal behavior masked by its pretensions to being a political movement. They were the first to attempt to alert the world to the nature of the rough slouching toward Berlin." And they kept up their brave journalistic resistance "for a dozen years." Hitler was obsessed with the defiant newspaper because "they knew how to get to him, get under his skin."

The newspaper nicknamed "the Poison Kitchen" might never have stood a chance to prevail, but its writers and editors persisted in the face of the darkening political situation of Hitler's rise to power. Rosenbaum noted, "It was an unfair, unseen struggle. They were a small band of scribblers taking on a well-financed army of murderous thugs. But in ways large and small, they made his life miserable." The newspaper consistently referred to the Nazi party as "the Hitler Party," because "their repeated use of the term was a relentless reminder to their readers that the crimes they reported on by Nazi Party members were the personal responsibility of one man, that the party they reported on was less a serious, ideologically based movement than an instrument of one man's criminal pathology." The heroic reporters, "men such as Martin Gruber, Erhard Auer, Edmund Goldshagg, Julius Zertass, among others—were in the trenches every day, taking on Hitler, facing down his thugs and their threats, testing the power of truth to combat evil, and sharing the Cassandra-like fate of discovering its limits." That "Poison Kitchen" of a newspaper showed the power of great journalism to peer into the future. According to Rosenbaum, the journalists of the *Munich Post* "even glimpsed through a glass darkly, the shadow of the Final Solution. In fact, they picked up the fateful Hitler euphemism for genocide—*endlösung*, the final solution—in the context of the fate of the Jews as early as December 9, 1931, in a chilling and prophetic dispatch called 'the Jews in the Third Reich.' " The *Munich Post* correctly saw the Nazi Party "as a homicidal criminal enterprise beneath the façade of a political party." Rosenbaum writes that, in the end, as their fate and the fate of Germany became clear, they had to accept "the shocking, crushing realization that despite their best efforts, their sacrifices, the years of struggle against Hitler, the ridicule, the exposés, the crimes, the death toll they pinned on him, Hitler had won—and all he'd threatened was about to come horrifically true." According to Rosenbaum, the *Munich Post* fought to the bitter end. Rosenbaum explained that his goal in writing about the *Munich Post* was "to restore the Poison Kitchen vision to historians whose attempts to explore Hitler could not help but benefit from exposure to the kind of investigative intimacy the *Munich Post* achieved in its hand-to-hand, eye-to-eye combat with [Hitler]."

It could be argued that if there was one "Poison Kitchen" during the AIDS and "chronic fatigue syndrome" epidemic, it was the *New York Native*. Although the newspaper was as unsuccessful as the *Munich Post* in preventing a human disaster of unprecedented scope, it at least put up a very determined fight, "hand to hand, eye-to-eye combat" with the political and pseudoscientific forces that gave the world the HIV/AIDS and "chronic fatigue syndrome is not AIDS" paradigms. The *New York Native* stood up week after week to the puppet masters of the catastrophe and, although the journalists of the *New York Native* did not suffer the same consequences as the journalists of the *Munich Post*, at the beginning of 1997, after fifteen years of being the AIDS and CFS establishment's "Poison Kitchen," the *New York Native,* was silenced.

1981-1984: The Fog of Epidemiology

News of what would eventually be called the AIDS epidemic first surfaced formally in the mass media in a shocking story in the *New York Times* on July 3, 1981, which I remember was an extremely hot day in Manhattan. I had left the *New York Native* office on West Fifty-seventh Street late and picked up an early edition of the *New York Times.* When I got home I was very tired but I was shaking by the time I finished reading the story. It would be one of those moments when time stood still, like the Kennedy assassination or the moment decades later when I turned on the TV the morning of 9/11. At the time I was the publisher and editor-in-chief of a struggling gay literary magazine called *Christopher Street* and *New York Native*, a gay paper that had been started the previous December in hopes of saving our struggling little publishing company. After reading the disturbing report about a supposedly mysterious cancer that was striking gay men, I immediately called the editor of both publications, Tom Steele, who had been working with me late at the office. My voice was quavering as I read him parts of the article. I didn't get much sleep that night.

In the ensuing days and weeks, I struggled to get ahold of the emerging amorphous facts about the mysterious new disease while grappling with the state of severe anxiety that the terrifying news had aroused in me. We asked a gay doctor we knew, Dr. Lawrence Mass, to investigate the cases—which were soon called "Gay-Related Immune Deficiency Syndrome"—for the paper. This was totally uncharted territory for me and we initially relied on Mass's medical background to help clarify what was going on for our readers. As I began to calm down and accept the situation we were in I soon chose a determined, pragmatic path for the newspaper. We would devote the paper to methodically getting to the bottom of the epidemic and make the disease the newspaper's signature story. While I was personally terrified of the implications, as a publisher I sensed that this was going to be a huge event. I tried to be optimistic. I told myself that in an age of scientific and technological genius and daily miracles surely a cause would be found and a cure would follow. Wasn't that how science operated?

In those early days, when what was initially labeled "Gay-Related Immune Deficiency" was evolving into "Acquired Immune Deficiency

Syndrome," a significant part of every business day was consumed with just trying to provide myself with the beginnings of a scientific education. English major, meet epidemiology, immunology and virology. Tom Steele had more of a scientific background than I did and he helped me familiarize myself with the workings of the immune system which seemed to be going awry in the gay victims of the epidemic. In that early period of the epidemic scientists noticed first that specific disease fighting cells in the immune system, namely T-cells, were not functioning or were decimated in gay men. Many gay men started going to their doctors to find out whether anything was wrong with their T-cells, and to my chagrin, at the time it seemed like everyone I talked to, who had a T-cell test, found out that they were suffering from a T-cell deficiency. It was hard at the time not to wonder apocalyptically if they all were going to get this disease and die. Unfortunately, it was mostly *gay* American men who were suddenly looking closely and suspiciously at their immune systems. If the whole country had followed suit, history might have turned out differently. Had we known about the so-called chronic fatigue syndrome epidemic at that point, we would have been talking about gay men as having an extreme or acute form of the immune dysfunction that had been seen in the chronic fatigue syndrome patients.

From 1981 to early in 1983, every kind of scientific hypothesis in the world was discussed as the possible cause of AIDS. As a publisher eager to know every possibility and to share them with the readers of *New York Native*, I was willing to listen to anyone who had an idea. I felt that the right answer could come from anywhere. Some people thought that AIDS was caused by recreational drug use. The director of the Centers for Disease Control's AIDS task force made a remark that he *hoped* it was poppers (amyl or butyl nitrite), a drug then heavily used by gay men to enhance sex. The drug causes the constriction of blood vessels and makes the heart beat faster, so that an orgasm is much more intense. But the CDC was unable to find a perfect correlation between the use of poppers and the mysterious disease. The same lack of correlation held true for other drugs that were then being used by gay men. The CDC also could not correlate any specific sexually transmitted disease with the array of symptoms which they had labeled "AIDS."

During those first two years of the epidemic, I was generally trustful of our government and the CDC scientists initially assigned to the problem. They seemed sincere and decent. When I talked to CDC scientists like James Curran, they seemed responsive and respectful. The scientists I had contact with did not strike me as being particularly anti-gay, although disconcerting AIDS jokes were beginning to circulate, even among physicians and scientists. I hoped they were not a sign of things to come.

Alarmingly, the cases began to mount and Lawrence Mass thoroughly covered each disturbing development that basically kept gay men in a permanent state of dread, always waiting for the next shoe to drop. As our reporting on the epidemic took up more and more space in *New York Native*, the circulation started to go down. Many people in the New York gay community wanted me to downplay the epidemic because they felt it was bad for the image of gay people and disastrous for gay businesses. One prominent businessman who spent a great deal of money advertising in the *Native* told me he was considering leaving the paper if we continued to cover the epidemic. I was concerned about the community's business—and the *Native*'s—but I felt it was the paper's responsibility to cover the story and to get to the bottom of it. To borrow a notion from Hannah Arendt, I felt like world history had broken out and *New York Native* was destined to play a part in the thick of it. I even fantasized that *New York Native* might play a significant role in ending the epidemic.

At one business meeting early in the epidemic, two of my advertising salespeople, Derek and Daniel, implored me to cut down on the coverage of the epidemic or at least keep it off the cover of *New York Native*. I told them that was not possible and that they would both have to try harder to sell ads. Within four years they were both dead from AIDS.

Frankly, *New York Native* did not have much of a skeptical or even investigative attitude towards the government during those first two years. A dramatic example of the paper's misplaced trust occurred when the director of the National Gay and Lesbian Task Force, Virginia Apuzzo, expressed some concern about confidentiality with regard to some AIDS research that was going on. I wrote an editorial suggesting that gay men would have to share information about their health to enable scientists in their search for the cause of the epidemic. I was assuming everything was being done in good faith in those days. Patients, doctors, scientists, the gay community, the government, we were all in it together. Supposedly.

In 1982, there was one thing that happened that did start to make me wonder about the government's role and integrity. There was a report that had nothing to do with AIDS directly, but was about two government agencies sharing the names of gay men in a variety of studies. It suggested that the government was playing fast and loose with gay privacy issues. I began to wonder if the CDC might be capable of similar questionable antics.

On March 14, 1983, I published what would turn out to be the most talked about piece—and most consequential—in the *New York Native's* history. At 5,000 words it was also the longest. "1,112 and Counting," by screenwriter and novelist Larry Kramer, appeared prominently on the cover and many now consider it the cri de coeur that launched (for better or worse) the era of AIDS activism.

Looking back three decades later at the piece, what I am most struck by is the way it captured the terror and the panic and the sense of impending catastrophe and doom in the gay community. At the time I was committed to making the pages of the *Native* available to any writer who would make a credible attempt to explain politically or scientifically what was going on or offer ideas on how to deal with the disaster that seemed to be growing exponentially on a daily basis.

Kramer began the article, "If this doesn't scare the shit out of you we're in real trouble. If this article doesn't rouse you to anger, fury, rage and action, gay men may have no future on earth. Our continued existence depends on just how angry you can get."

His call for anger and more anger would turn out over the years to be boilerplate Kramer. One person with chronic fatigue syndrome told me years later that she approached Kramer after one of his public jeremiads and said, "Mr. Kramer, I just want to thank you for your anger." Over the years urging people *to be angry* began to strike me as a very peculiar gospel.

Throughout his piece Kramer portrayed the gay community as being on the brink of extinction. He presented the current numbers of dead and dying and left the impression of a tsunami of a plague that might engulf every gay man in its path. He wrote, "For the first time in the epidemic, leading doctors and researchers are finally admitting they don't know what is going on." His parade of horribles included a doctor who was sorry he ever got involved with the mysterious disease, packed hospitals, patients being treated as "lepers," and gay suicides in the face of the horror. He spoke of an outrageous lack of funding for research, blaming it on anti-gay prejudice. He wrote that the straight medical community which supposedly knew the disease was not going to stay limited to gays could "use us as guinea pigs to discover the cure for AIDS before it hits them, which most medical authorities are still convinced will be happening shortly in increasing numbers." And use "us" they ultimately did.

Kramer took a shot at the man who would become his personal bête noire: New York City's Mayor Ed Koch. He wrote, "Repeated attempts to meet with him have been denied us. Repeated attempts to have him make a very necessary public announcement about this crisis and public health emergency have been refused by his staff." He complained about the mayor's liaison to the gay community, Herb Rickman, basically portraying him as a gay enemy of the gay community, someone who was incompetent and insensitive to the political needs of the hour.

In a litany of things Kramer was "sick of," he listed elected officials "who in no way represent us," "closeted gay doctors," "closeted gays," "guys who moan that giving up careless sex until this blows over is worse than death," "guys who think that all being gay means is sex in the first place," and "every gay man who does not get behind this issue totally and with commitment—to fight for his life." We didn't realize at the time the degree to which that getting behind this issue meant getting behind Kramer and his poorly grounded epidemiological beliefs and rage-driven rhetoric.

Kramer criticized "the *Advocate*, the country's largest gay publication, which has yet to quite acknowledge that there's anything going on . . . . And their own associate editor, Brent Harris, died from AIDS." He wrote, "With the exception of the *Native*, and a few, very few other gay publications, the gay press has been useless."

What he said about the Centers for Disease Control in the piece is quite ironic, given what was to come to light in the next three decades. He wrote, "If there have been—and there may have been—any cases in straight, white non-intravenous drug-using, middle-class Americans, the Centers for Disease Control isn't telling anyone about them. . . . The CDC also tends not to believe white, middle-class male victims when they say they say they're straight, or female victims when they say their husbands are straight and don't take drugs." Regardless of his criticism of the CDC's competence, its funding, or its ability to keep up with the expanding caseload, there really wasn't much daylight between the CDC's epidemiological presumptions about what AIDS was and how it was transmitted—and the "careless sex" notions that were implicit and explicit in Kramer's historic rant. And every other piece he vented in during the next three decades.

One red flag about Kramer's addled political judgment that stands out in his piece is this statement: "Southern newspapers and Jerry Falwell's publications are already printing editorials proclaiming AIDS as God's deserved punishment to homosexuals. So what? Nasty words make poor little sissy pansy wilt and die?"

He ended the article with the names of twenty-one people he knew (some with just first names) who had died of the illness and closed with, "If we don't act immediately, then we face our approaching doom."

In the same issue, Larry Bush reported on a development that certainly would give "poor little sissy pansies" pause. Margaret Heckler was about to become the Secretary of Health and Human Services. Bush wrote, "Heckler had served in Congress for 16 years before being defeated by Rep. Barney Frank (D. Mass.) in last fall's general election. Frank received the largest single contribution from the Human Rights Campaign Fund in 1982, partly because he was matched for re-election against a woman who had voted to deny gays access to federal legal services and to retain the ten-year prison term provided for sodomy convictions in Washington, D.C."

Shortly after we published the Kramer piece, I received a phone call from John Berendt, then an editor at *Geo* magazine. He had just read an interesting hypothesis about the cause of AIDS in *New Scientist*, a colorful British scientific journal that is a mixture of serious and "pop" science. The brief article was about a letter that had been published in one of the world's leading medical journals, *The Lancet*. In the letter a young scientist in Boston named Jane Teas proposed for the first time that AIDS might be caused by African swine fever virus. She pointed out that the symptoms of AIDS closely resembled those of African swine fever. She also noted that in Haiti, which also had a growing AIDS epidemic, there was simultaneously an epidemic of African swine fever virus in pigs. She hypothesized that vacationing gay men might have contracted the disease by eating undercooked pork.

I instantly thought the theory was reasonable and should be explored. It had the ring of truth to it. I discussed the hypothesis with James D'Eramo, a man with a Ph.D. in medical ecology and infectious diseases, who had become our new science reporter, and I asked him to call Teas and arrange to interview her in Boston, which he did the following weekend. I was feeling very competitive about the story. I wanted *New York Native* to publish the first lengthy interview with her.

When D'Eramo got back from Boston and filled me in on her ideas,

I was even more convinced that her hypothesis was the most compelling one I had heard in two years. We published his interview with Teas in the May 23, 1983, issue and started it on the cover with the headline, "Is African Swine Fever the Cause?"

The day the article appeared, something weird happened. A gay activist in New York attacked the idea publicly and said he thought the Teas idea was racist. That struck me as very strange and I wondered if we had hit some mysterious political nerve. It wasn't the reaction I was expecting from anyone in the gay community.

At the time that Teas wrote her letter, she was a postgraduate student at the Harvard School of Public Health and she didn't have much money. I was soon talking to her on a regular basis and she told me she wished she could attend a conference in Florida about exotic animal diseases because some sessions of the meeting were going to focus on African swine fever. I offered to pay for the trip to the conference because I was convinced the scientists there might support her idea and help test it.

She called us after the first day of the conference and was elated. She had presented her ideas at one of the African swine fever sessions. When she was done, the man who was leading the session denounced her idea to the audience, but afterwards, a number of scientists approached her and expressed their enthusiasm about the idea that there was a link between African swine fever and AIDS. She began to make arrangements at the conference to test her hypothesis with some of the scientists. At that point I thought the money to send her there had been well spent.

But that all changed later that week. She called to tell us that at a reception near the end of the conference, she had seen the interested scientists talking to government officials who were in attendance. Subsequently, one by one, the scientists who had previously been enthusiastic about her idea approached her to tell her they would not be able to investigate her hypothesis. She felt that they had all been pressured to change their minds.

From the very beginning of the epidemic, government scientists had given the impression that finding out what was the cause of AIDS was their first and only priority. It therefore puzzled me when there was government resistance about testing Teas's very reasonable African swine fever hypothesis. When Jane Teas wrote directly to the CDC in April of 1983 to explain her ASFV idea, she received a cold shoulder. Dr. Michael Gregg, the deputy director of the Epidemiology

Program Office, wrote to Teas that he had shared her thoughts with Dr. James Curran (of the AIDS Task Force) and Dr. John Bennett, Assistant Director for Medical Science at the Center for Infectious Diseases. Gregg wrote back to Teas, "Rest assured that if they and other members of the senior staff here feel that more effort should be directed to uncover any real association between [AIDS and African swine fever], it will be done. As I believe I implied in our telephone conversation, it is relatively difficult for outside scientists such as yourself to impact directly on research programs within a center such as CDC. Quite frankly, perhaps the best you can expect is an acknowledgement with thanks. Nevertheless, I do wish to convey to you my personal thanks for your obvious interest and encouragement. As you state, the power of the pen should not be underestimated." In retrospect, this looks like the elitist don't-bother-us attitude that is typical of the hermetically sealed world of abnormal science that AIDS turned out to be.

On May 14, 1983, the first scientific rebuttal to Teas's hypothesis appeared in *The Lancet*. Five European researchers signed a letter that indicated that they had tested hospital patients with AIDS for antibodies to African swine fever virus. They reported that none of the patients were positive. However, they did leave a door open: "Attempts at ASFV antigen demonstration and at growing the elusive AIDS agent in swine cells supporting ASFV isolation could be made to investigate further the ASFV hypothesis in AIDS patients. Our results, however, make it unlikely that ASFV and the AIDS agent will be found to be related." Teas was dissatisfied with their approach and felt that their negative findings were questionable.

That same month, Gary Noble, the Acting Director of the Division of Viral Diseases at the CDC, sent a memo to his colleagues noting, "Considerable interest in the possible role of African swine fever virus (ASFV) has been generated by Dr. Jane Teas's letter to *The Lancet* . . . . Although no known human infection with ASFV has ever occurred, the presence of ASFV infection among swine in Haiti and the ability of the virus to induce some immunosuppression among pigs has led to the hypothesis proposed by Dr. Teas of the Harvard School of Public Health. . . . We have received calls from Dr. Sheldon Landesman, Director, AIDS Haitian Study Group, Downstate Medical Center, New York, asking if we would test sera from Haitians with and without AIDS. Dr. Fred Siegel, Director of Medicine, Mt. Sinai School of Medicine, has offered to send sera from AIDS patients for testing for ASFV antibodies. We have also been asked by Jane Teas and Lawrence Altman, *New York Times*, if we proposed to do testing for sera from AIDS patients for antibodies to ASFV."

Noble then added that the Department of Agriculture had shipped the CDC materials necessary to test AIDS sera for antibodies to ASFV and he made some suggestions about how the testing should be done.

In June, a very odd letter appeared in *The Lancet* in response to the Teas hypothesis. It was written by Ronald K. St. John of the Epidemiology Unit of the Pan American Health Organization. He wrote that he took issue with her hypothesis of a "possible cycle for the accidental introduction of ASFV into the human population. She speculates that, through an improbable series of events, AIDS originated in Haiti. There is no epidemiological evidence to support the ideas. Allegations, without strong supporting epidemiological evidence, that one country is responsible for introducing an illness are reminiscent of syphilis in the Middle Ages, when the French worried about the 'Italian disease,' and vice versa."

St. John wrote, "Investigation in Haiti by the Haitian Ministry of Health, the Pan American Health Organization (PAHO), and the U.S. Department of Agriculture indicated that African swine fever is not being transmitted from pigs to man, and for these and other reasons it seems unlikely that it could be the cause of AIDS."

Tragically, Teas's hypothesis was being totally distorted. She wasn't blaming Haiti. She was just suggesting that a relatively unsurprising zoonotic event may have occurred there. Pigs have a lot in common with humans and it is hardly shocking to think that a disease other than the flu could come from pigs. If her idea was correct it could have had the effect of saving many lives in Haiti itself.

I began to realize that ASFV was an emotionally loaded and very political issue. Suddenly AIDS had become a matter that involved international relations. I started wondering how, in such a rancorous, hypersensitive environment, the search for truth could proceed in earnest. I didn't realize that the environment would turn into a virtual minefield for anyone with an open mind who dared to get involved in the years that followed.

A month later, on July 9, in *The Lancet*, several scientists attempted to put the matter completely to rest. Curiously, they reported that in December, 1982, before Jane Teas had even sent her idea to *The Lancet*, they "looked for antibody to ASFV in serum from Haitian patients with AIDS. In the serum of eight patients and four normal controls there was no evidence of antibody to ASFV." At the very least they clearly had shared her epidemiological suspicions about ASFV. The letter ended on what was becoming a rather familiar political note: "The hypothesis that AIDS originated in Haiti . . . is damaging to Haiti and to Haitian communities abroad." What they didn't mention is that the hypothesis, if confirmed, was also potentially damaging to the multibillion dollar pork industry in America and all over the world.

From the first day I heard about ASFV, I made an effort to get my hands on every article ever written about the wily and devastating virus. At the time there were over a thousand written about ASFV which had been discovered in 1909 by a Dr. Montgomery. For a while African swine fever was called Montgomery's disease. The more I read about ASFV, the more the porcine disease matched aspects of AIDS that had emerged in the early research. As new data was published on AIDS I kept comparing the findings to what was known about ASFV and the Teas hypothesis became more and more credible. Soon I had a sheet of paper with a list of twenty symptoms or immune problems that AIDS and African swine fever had in common. The cavalier and dismissive way the idea was being treated by AIDS researchers and the government increasingly seemed odd and irrational.

After the first response to her hypothesis was published, Teas wrote to *The Lancet*, noting that the experiment conducted by the European scientists "has not definitively disproved my idea." She pointed out that the scientists had not established which strain of the virus they utilized. She also noted that the antigen used in the test was irradiated (a process through which live virus is subjected to levels of radiation that render it harmless), which could have reduced the sensitivity of the test. She also argued that the clinical status of the patients could have affected the ability of the scientists to detect the presence of antibodies to the virus. She also warned that there is often a decline in circulating antibodies in pigs late in an ASFV infection. She ended her letter by describing the biggest problem in researching the possible link between AIDS and African swine fever: "The near impossibility of obtaining ASFV antigen in the continental United States and the reluctance of the United States Department of Agriculture at Plum Island [New York] to study human pathogens shrouds the question of an ASFV-AIDS link in unnecessary mystery." What Teas didn't know is that she had gotten herself involved in the opposite world of abnormal science which is always shrouded "in unnecessary mystery." Or worse.

At the time, all research on African swine fever had to be either performed on Plum Island, a small island off the coast of Long Island, New York, or it had to be conducted using virus that is irradiated in order to prevent accidental outbreak of African swine fever on the mainland of the United States. The USDA lived in mortal fear of an ASFV epidemic which, if it ever spread across the United States, in addition to destroying the pork business overnight, could become a permanent fixture because there is no treatment, no vaccine, and the virus can infect ticks and become endemic. Unfortunately, the dangerousness of the virus gave the government almost absolute power over the act of researching it on the mainland of the United States. There could basically be no research on ASFV without the willing participation—and oversight—of the American government.

Other scientists and lay people were beginning to take an interest in the possible connection. Fred Maurer, a retired veterinarian who had conducted extensive research on African swine fever virus in Africa, wrote to James Curran at the CDC, "Having worked with African swine fever virus (ASFV) for several years in Africa and on the pathology of it here, I fully agree with the possible relationship made by Jane Teas." He suggested that a pig be inoculated with the blood of a febrile AIDS patient, because "the remarkable similarity of the infection relative to the destruction of the immune system and the rapid mutation potential of the ASF virus, surely make such a study worth doing."

The CDC began to test the AIDS-ASFV hypothesis in June. Memos obtained by the *Native* that were written by Gary Noble, the Acting Director of the Division of Viral diseases, indicated that they planned to search for African swine fever virus in AIDS tissue samples using antisera provided by the U.S. Department of Agriculture. A Brooklyn doctor sent the CDC blood from ten Haitians with AIDS and five non-Haitians with AIDS, as well as additional blood from healthy Haitian controls. The CDC also planned to send some of the blood to Spain to be tested by African swine fever experts there.

A memo I obtained about the testing from the CDC, which was signed by "Paul," who was probably Paul Feorino, a lab worker who was involved in the testing, stated, "We must finish off the ASFV issue." His word choice beautifully captured the CDC's attitude toward the hypothesis.

I called the CDC frequently all that summer to try and find out what the results were. Late that summer, I was told by AIDS researcher

Donald Francis that the results were negative. At that point I thought the matter was dead and African swine fever had no involvement in AIDS. Case closed.

But things changed dramatically in the fall.

Earlier that summer, I had been in touch with Susan Steinmetz, a legislative aide to Congressman Ted Weiss of Manhattan. Weiss served on a committee that had, among other things, the responsibility of overseeing the activities of the Centers for Disease Control. As Weiss's assistant, Steinmetz helped audit the activities of the CDC and during a visit to the CDC offices in the autumn, she accidentally happened upon a memo on the results of the African swine fever testing and knowing I was interested, she sent me a copy. The results as reported on the ASFV memo couldn't exactly be described as negative. Out of ninety different blood samples from AIDS patients and controls, five showed some degree of positivity for African swine fever virus. Two of the CDC's ten control samples were positive, as well as three of the sixteen AIDS patients from San Francisco. Around that same time, I learned that the USDA had tested 47 members of its staff at Plum Island for antibodies to ASFV and 6 had tested positive.

What all of this told me was that the matter was not closed at all and that additional research would be appropriate. I called Jane Teas and told her that I felt that Francis had misinformed us. I also called Don Francis and confronted him with what was in the memo. He told me that because some of the controls were positive, he had made a *judgment call* that there was no relationship between AIDS and African swine fever. I had met Francis at one of the first major AIDS conferences in New York City the year before and I had listened to him talk at a reception later at Leonard Bernstein's apartment. Francis has struck me as arrogant and pompous, and unlike most of the assembled (mostly gay) guests, I was decidedly *not* impressed by him. Even though he was slightly older than myself, he seemed young and cocky and the last person whose judgment call should be taken as the final word on something as important as the cause of AIDS. It was chilling to me to think that this character had the power to make such fateful decisions.

In August of 1983, Jane Teas had written a two-page letter to Senator Durenberger of Minnesota, in which she asked for help in pursuing her ASFV hypothesis further. She complained that the negative letters published in *The Lancet* gave "no information . . . on the patients, and in addition, almost no information is given on the source of the antigen, the type of antigen used, or details of the tests employed." She underlined the political issues she feared were impeding thorough research: "Clearly the USDA is worried that the pig farmers may get upset, and the Pan American Health Organization is worried that I and the boat people, as well as the Haitian AIDS patients, are giving Haiti a bad name. However, it remains that at least 160 Haitians in Haiti have AIDS, and that there have been no reported cases from other Caribbean resort areas also frequented by gay American vacationers. To declare that Haiti is blameless seems irrelevant in trying to trace the cause of AIDS. With more than 2,000 AIDS patients, a more complete study of this association between a suddenly low virulent strain of ASFV and a suddenly appearing human disease is warranted."

On August 29, 1983, Durenberger forwarded the Teas letter to the CDC and requested that information on the inquiry be sent to his office. On September 23, Dr. William Foege wrote back to Durenberger's office, "ASFV does not appear to play any role in AIDS. With the help of virologists at Plum Island, the Centers for Disease Control has performed tests on serum from AIDS patients using target cells infected with ASFV. No positive reactions have been observed from AIDS patients' serum. In addition, CDC has used methods similar to those used to grow ASFV from pigs to culture circulating blood cells from over 100 people including patients with AIDS, patients with lymphadenopathy, and healthy contacts of AIDS patients. No cytopathic effect or other signs of ASFV have been detected. Although work continues, there is no laboratory evidence to confirm an etiologic link between ASFV and AIDS, as suggested by Dr. Teas. CDC, the Food and Drug Administration, and others have concluded that such a link is extremely unlikely."

On October 14, 1983, Durenberger forwarded the letter to Teas, and though she was unhappy with the response, she didn't write again to Durenberger until January 24, 1984. She thanked him and told him that she had thought the matter was closed but that "the *New York Native* editor, Chuck Ortleb sent me copies of CDC memos which clearly state that there were at least some positive for ASFV in the samples they tested. Dr. Donald Francis appears to have given incorrect information to Dr. Foege . . . with regard to the results of the CDC test, [and] the tests at Plum Island, where 6/47 workers were positive for ASF. . .."

She also told Durenberger that I had pressured the CDC to do more testing, which I had done through a series of phone calls and editorials in the *Native*. Teas asked for Durenberger's help in getting the Secretary of Agriculture's assistance, because his cooperation was required for the CDC to do additional research on African swine fever. She also outlined her plans to take this matter to scientists outside the United States: "In disgust, and after being told it was necessary to go outside of this country to have my theory tested, I have turned to research institutes outside of this country. However, in both England and South Africa, officials have told me that it is illegal to study African swine fever virus, they have no experience with AIDS and/or no experience with African swine fever virus." She then expressed a concern that if AIDS was indeed caused by African swine fever virus, then it was only a matter of time before all of the American pigs and all the pork products were infected with the virus, thus endangering every American who came in contact with undercooked pork. What she didn't know was that, unbeknownst to AIDS researchers, at that very time an AIDS-like illness *was indeed* spreading throughout the pig population in parts of North America.

By the beginning of 1984, I had become extremely concerned about the games that the CDC and the Department of Agriculture seemed to playing with the Teas ASFV/AIDS hypothesis. I tried something I had done before in *New York Native*. I wrote an editorial in the form of an open letter. This one was addressed to James Mason, Director of the CDC, John Block, the Secretary of Agriculture, Edward Brandt, the Director of the National Institutes of Health, and Lawrence Altman, a medical reporter for the *New York Times* (and ex-CDC employee) who was covering AIDS. I included Altman because of the paltry coverage he had given in the *Times* to the Teas hypothesis. In general, he seemed to just parrot whatever the government said about the AIDS issue. Here is the text of the open letter:

Dear Gentlemen:

As our readers know, this paper has provided more diverse and up-to-date information about AIDS than any other non-medical publication in America. Even at the risk of being labeled "The New York Native Journal of Medicine," we have consistently tried to stay on top of the AIDS story, which we continue to feel is the biggest medical story of the Eighties. We have provided information on the results of all kinds of research. We have given every theory its day in the sun, and we still don't know *what* causes AIDS. From where we sit, we see all kinds of work going on in appropriate areas; most hypotheses have at least some degree of funding and adequate personnel working on them. Still nothing looks terribly promising, although we've been told privately that more encouraging news may soon emerge from the French team who discovered LAV (Lymphadenopathy Associated Virus).

Yet one thing continues to puzzle us: the resistance that has confronted pathobiologist Jane Teas's hypothesis that African swine fever virus is the cause of AIDS. And some recent information with which the *Native* has been presented has us even more puzzled.

Apparently, back in June, the Centers for Disease Control tested some AIDS sera for antibodies to African swine fever virus. Virologist Dr. Donald Francis, who is coordinator of AIDS laboratory activities, told us a few months later that the results were "negative." We were interested in studying exactly how the tests were performed, and we asked Dr. Francis if he intended to write up the methods and results for a medical journal. Dr. Francis told us that the CDC could not get much done if it went about publishing all its negative results. Perhaps, but negative results did not prevent the CDC from publishing the outcome of its analysis of receptive anal intercourse as a risk factor for developing AIDS. (If only African swine fever virus involved some sexual act which would capture the prurient imaginations of the CDC and the NIH, we'd have some thorough testing— pronto.)

When Dr. Francis told us about the African swine fever test results and his intention not to write up the results for publication, we probably should have been a good little gay newspaper and politely withdrawn without asking any further questions. Instead, we tracked down the CDC memorandum that described some of this testing. It turns out that "negative" is not exactly the report given by the memorandum. . . . Out of over 50 sera tested, two of the controls and two of the AIDS sera apparently showed some degree of positivity. The controls were from the CDC staff. (One researcher with whom we discussed the methods remarked that the CDC staff sera might not be the best of controls in such testing.) The fact that two of the controls tested positive contributed to Dr. Francis's judgment that all the positives were false positive. If Dr. Francis had been an experienced African swine fever virus researcher, he probably would have performed 11 further conventional tests just to verify his results. Any positivity should cause enough alarm to generate further testing. To the best of our understanding . . . a plan was subsequently devised to do additional testing with "whole [ASFV] virus from Plum Island." At the same time, Dr. Francis was apparently having the AIDS sera tested to determine whether African swine fever virus had a cytopathic (cell-killing) effect on human lymphocytes. (It is possible that the modified form of African swine fever virus is non-cytopathic and non-hemadsorbing. Sorry if that's too technical; please keep reading.) There was no cytopathic effect found.

Meanwhile, back at Plum Island (which is a USDA testing center off the coast of Long Island), a messy little situation had developed. They were also testing their own staff's blood for antibodies to African swine fever virus, and, lo and behold, six of the staff tested positive. The test they used is called the E.L.I.S.A. test, and it is touted as one of the most sensitive (with no more than a one percent false positive.) Out of the total number of sera tested, 20 percent were positive. Again, because some of those tested had no exposure (so far as they knew) to African swine fever virus, they assumed that these were false positive results, and they did one additional test to make sure. The results, as far as we know, were kept secret from the staff and the rest of the world. When one of the world experts on African swine fever virus who works at Plum Island was told by the *Native* about the results of the tests, he was quite upset that he hadn't been informed by his associates. When he confronted one of his associates about the results, the response was, "How did you find that out?" Well, a gay newspaper told him, of course. The secrecy that surrounds this testing just adds a little more spice to the mystery of the story.

Meanwhile, back at the CDC, plans were being made to send AIDS sera to Madrid for testing for African swine fever virus. They could just as easily have been sent to Plum Island, which is quite capable of doing the testing. That was in June.

When we confronted CDC Drs. James Curran, Fred Murphy, and Don Francis with the memoranda that we had seen, the story of AIDS and African swine fever changed a bit. Now Dr. Curran describes the tests as "inconclusive." Dr. Murphy describes the tests as "incomplete." When we asked Dr. Francis if the CDC had the results from the June tests from Madrid, we were told that they did not. We offered to call Madrid if the CDC was too busy to bother. We were told that "maybe they're having the same problem with their test that we're having." Yes, true positives or false positives would be a problem. Especially true positives.

The point to all of this is that the possibility still remains that African swine fever virus is the cause of AIDS. The CDC may have already given the first indication of that without realizing it. In any case, Dr. Francis should not be giving the scientific community the impression that the results of the CDC testing of this hypothesis are a good reason for them to dismiss it.

The whole matter could be regarded from another perspective. The United States Department of Agriculture has the major responsibility of making sure that African swine fever virus is not present in any animal (human or otherwise) in this country. It is absurd for the USDA to put anyone in the position of begging that agency to do its job. One of their fraternity, Dr. Fred Maurer, a respected Doctor of Veterinary

Medicine and a Ph.D. who has worked with African swine fever virus in Africa, has notified the USDA that he thinks there is a strong possibility that AIDS is caused by ASFV. Dr. Jerry Callis, the director of the Plum Island facilities, has a responsibility to take this matter seriously for the sake of all the farmers he is supposed to be protecting from African swine fever virus. Dr. James Mason, the director of the CDC, has a responsibility to take this matter seriously for the sake of all the American he is supposed to be protecting from AIDS.

As a result of the letter, I received a call from Don Berreth, the director of the press office of the CDC. He told me that the director of the CDC was coming to New York in April and that he wanted to meet with me. I became optimistic that we could talk the CDC into doing additional research on the possible African swine fever connection when we met with Mason.

Meanwhile, it appeared that we had made enough noise to force the CDC to give the appearance of taking the ASFV hypothesis seriously. Over and over we had argued that the strongest and most direct way to investigate the hypothesis would be to inoculate healthy pigs with blood from someone with AIDS. The seriousness with which the CDC took this idea was reflected in a memo dated December 1983 from Frederick Murphy, Director of the Division of Viral Diseases at CDC. Sent to Don Francis, the memo outlined their plan: "Per telephone conversation with Dr. J. J. Callis, Director, Plum Island Center (P.I.A.D.C.) on 13 December, it was agreed to proceed with planning toward conducting an experiment at Plum Island (under P-4) conditions wherein swine would be inoculated with materials from AIDS patients. This experiment would provide final resolutions of the premise still being made publicly that AIDS is caused by ASFV virus. Final decision as to the feasibility of doing this experiment will be made by Dr. Callis shortly." (This porcine AIDS experiment, which was supposed to put the matter to rest, *was never done*.)

I had several conversations about African swine fever virus with Callis in which he was consistently contemptuous about the very notion that AIDS was *anything at all* like African swine fever. I had come close to having verbal fisticuffs with him on one occasion. His personal field of expertise was hoof-and-mouth disease. I was disturbed by the fact that he told me things about African swine fever that I knew from my survey of the scientific literature were absolutely false. He insisted that ASFV is not a very changeable virus even though the whole history of this virus, which was discovered in 1909, is characterized by dramatic and insidious changes in virulence. When it was first discovered, it killed over 97 percent of pigs infected, but, by the time it hit Haiti, in 1976, it was killing less than 3 percent of the pigs it infected. Its characteristic symptoms had evolved from severe hemorrhaging to symptoms like pneumonia, arthritis, and motor disturbances. I thought that either Callis was deliberately lying or was surprisingly stupid. He was clearly miffed that he was being forced by lay people to deal with this hypothesis. No doubt the fact that this whole affair was being driven by a gay newspaper made the matter even more unpleasant for him.

Throughout this period, I tried to get other newspapers interested in the story. I didn't want the issue ghettoized in our little newspaper. I didn't want to own the story. That was a formula for credibility disaster. I made contact with a local newspaper on Long Island that served the area near Plum Island and convinced a reporter to do a story about the planned testing. A CDC memo from Don Francis noted that Callis called Francis to tell him that the local press was "breaking a story on Plum Island doing AIDS research." The memo also stated, "Callis is reluctant about having potentially infectious [AIDS] sera at Plum Island and does not want sera to be irradiated and is going to suggest CDC do the testing." Even though Plum Island worked with the most dangerous animal viruses, Callis was concerned about having AIDS sera there. That's how scary AIDS was in those days.

Callis sent a memo to the nearly 300 employees who worked on Plum Island: "A letter by Jane Teas of the Harvard School of Public Health, published in the journal *Lancet*, April 23, 1983, speculated that since AIDS occurred in Haitians and African swine fever also appeared in Haiti, AIDS might be caused by African swine fever (ASF) virus. Most who are knowledgeable of ASF have rejected this supposition, including medical authorities in Haiti. Swine ill from ASF show very little clinical similarity to AIDS in men. Also those who have worked with ASF virus or have lived in areas where the disease has existed for long periods of time have not become ill because of this contact. In spite of the overwhelming evidence that these are different diseases, the hypothesis may require testing. Thus, discussions are continuing with scientists from the Centers for Disease Control (CDC) in Atlanta, and they may request such work be undertaken under controlled conditions in secure animal facilities so that ASF virus may be used in the studies required. It is federal policy that all agencies of the government will assist each other as circumstances dictate as described above."

On March 1, 1984, the CDC's Don Francis wrote a memo describing a conference call with Callis and Dr. Kenneth Cell of the National Institutes of Allergy and Infectious Diseases. He noted, "Although there was strong serologic and virologic evidence against any association between ASFV and AIDS, some further testing was necessary to confirm previous results." The memo outlined plans for additional serological testing that would be more sophisticated than the original testing performed by the CDC. It also noted that Dr. William Hess, a swine fever expert with whom I had been speaking several times each week, would come to the CDC to work with Dr. Paul Feorino in conducting tests. Francis also wrote, "Following the results of these serologic tests, further consideration will be given to injecting pigs with AIDS material at Plum Island." (Again, *that was never done*.)

Teas, D'Eramo, and I were very concerned that the new testing still might not be sophisticated enough to settle the matter. D'Eramo wrote to Mason, giving him suggestions on how to perform the tests so that the results would not likely be challenged. D'Eramo emphasized that it was important that AIDS sera be tested for a wide variety of strains of African swine fever virus. He noted that three different kinds of tests needed to be done just to reach a 90 percent level of confidence. He also urged the CDC to publish the results of the tests with a full description of the testing process. Most importantly, he strongly suggested, "Materials from CDC-defined AIDS cases and materials from ARC [AIDS-Related Complex] patients should be inoculated (with controls) into laboratory swine. This procedure may provide a satisfactory animal model for AIDS."

This all came to a crashing halt in April 1984, when D'Eramo and I met with CDC Director James Mason at the Health Department in Manhattan. Mason was a bland bureaucrat who didn't strike me as being the brightest bulb in the world during the forty-five minutes we spent with him. The CDC's press officer, Don Berreth, sat beside Mason, often qualifying his boss's statements. I implored Mason to contact African swine fever expert William Hess, who had been open-minded about an ASFV-AIDS connection in my discussions with him.

It was unfortunate and a bad sign that Mason kept referring to African swine fever as "Swine flu." At the meeting Mason told us that the CDC was about to announce that they knew what the cause of AIDS was: a retrovirus called Lymphadenopathy Associated Virus which had been discovered by the Pasteur Institute in Paris. I have been told by reporters that I should have been flattered that in essence we were being given privileged inside information. Journalists have found it ironic that at the very moment it became clear we were not going to get to first base with the CDC on ASF, we were actually being giving a world-class scoop by the director of the CDC. At the same time our concern about ASFV was being blown off, it simultaneously showed the uncanny power of the *Native*. It was the last moment in history when the *Native* had that kind of importance to the government or the AIDS establishment.

But when the whole world learned that the cause of AIDS had supposedly been found, it wasn't LAV, the virus Mason had told us about, that was celebrated. On April 23, 1984, Margaret Heckler, then Secretary of Health and Human Services, called a press conference in Washington, D.C. to announce, "The probable cause of AIDS has been found—a variant of a known human cancer virus, called HTLV-III." She also told the press that a test to screen the blood supply for the presence of this virus would be available in six months, and that a vaccine would be ready for testing in two years. The people she credited for the discovery included Robert Gallo, Dr. Edward Brandt (Assistant Secretary of Health), Dr. Vincent DeVita (Director of the National Cancer Institute), Drs. James Mason and James Curran of the CDC. She also pointed out the contributions of the French scientists had made—which would turn out to be the understatement of the century. Within a year the French and American scientists would be viciously fighting over the issue of who had actually discovered the so-called cause of AIDS.

The Heckler announcement was electrifying. Suddenly there was a light at the end of the terrifying AIDS tunnel. I had mixed feelings about the announcement because of my distrust of Gallo and his close associate at Harvard, retroviral researcher Dr. Myron Essex. A scientist named Larry Falk had approached Jane Teas after her letter had been published in *The Lancet* in 1983. At the time, Falk was one of Essex's collaborator's on HTLV-related AIDS research. He had suggested to Teas that perhaps the virus that Essex had found in AIDS patients was actually the form that African swine fever virus took in man, an extremely odd suggestion given that ASFV is a large DNA virus and the HTLVs are retroviruses. I was wary of the fact that Essex was a consultant to the USDA's Plum Island facility at the time when the USDA was being very uncooperative in testing the Teas ASFV hypothesis, which was certainly competitive with Essex's retroviral AIDS hypothesis. And then there was the disturbing moment when a leading AIDS researcher at St. Luke's Roosevelt Hospital in New York—one of the few who remained trustworthy over the three decades of the epidemic—said to me during the time that Gallo and Essex were originally trying to prove HTLV-I was the cause of AIDS, "You know, scientists in Europe consider Essex and Gallo to be crooks."

The *Native* was one of the first newspapers to do an extensive interview with Robert Gallo after the Heckler announcement. In the August 24, 1984, issue, James D'Eramo asked Gallo why he thought that "AIDS" had broken out in gay men and he replied, "Well it's not staying in the homosexual community anymore; now the virus has spread. I have the impression that there's too much attention paid to all the details of the sexual practices. There's too much interest in that." Ironically, Gallo may inadvertently have been onto the very issue of biased epidemiology, or what I have coined as "homodemiology," which had completely distorted the picture of "AIDS" with tragic consequences for the whole human race. It was almost as though Gallo, at least subconsciously, could see the real epidemic that lurked below the Potemkin epidemic of HIV (as HTLV-III eventually became known) when he said to D'Eramo, "What about normal healthy people with no disease symptoms at all who aren't sexually active, who are not IV-drug users—are they completely risk free? I don't think so. I think they're at risk of getting infected too. The virus just needs to grow in these populations."

Gallo could also have been unknowingly pointing to the real underlying pandemic when he said, "Rather than focusing per se on the nature of sexual practice, I believe this virus can be transmitted by any form of intimate contact. I don't care what it is." He went beyond the government's official epidemiological line when he said, "I don't think kissing on the cheek is a problem, but if you exchange saliva, you may be at risk."

At that point Gallo had dug his heels in on the issue of AIDS causation: "Clearly HTLV-III causes AIDS. Anybody who doesn't say that doesn't know the facts. There's no question about it. . . . I think there's more evidence that this is the cause of AIDS than there is on the majority of microbiological agents that you and I routinely accept as the cause of other diseases." Gallo might as well have declared that science was about to proudly march into the darkness and total domination of totalitarianism for the next three decades.

D'Eramo asked Gallo, "Do you think other viruses, like CMV or EBV, play a role in the development of AIDS? Dr. Jane Teas told us a long time ago about the idea of African swine fever virus coming from Africa to Haiti and then from Haiti to America." Gallo replied, "It turns out even though she had the wrong virus, she seems to have had the right idea about the origins of the virus."

When D'Eramo asked about HTLV-III fulfilling Koch's postulates (a set of traditional scientific rules for proving causation), Gallo basically pooh-poohed the idea: "We should remember we have progressed in some ways since that time. Some people don't seem to know that. For example, Robert Koch did not have modern microbiology or serology; he didn't have seroepidemiology." (Or, what I might have called sero*homo*demiology.)

Gallo insisted to D'Eramo that HTLV-III was not an opportunistic infection. He didn't think that anyone should look for any other cause.

When D'Eramo asked whether further experiments had been done to determine if Gallo's virus was the same as the Pasteur retrovirus, Gallo, true to character, went ballistic: "This is a question that is asked too much, and people don't even know why they're asking it anymore." He then told D'Eramo something that was later shown by *Chicago Tribune* reporter John Crewdson to be a lie: "I have 86 isolates of HTLV-III and I have shown that those 86 isolates are the same virus. We published 48 isolates at once."

About gay men, Gallo said, "I have heard there are some so seriously driven that they are like alcoholics . . . . Yes, I have that from Dr. Curran. There are some that are so hypersexual that they're like alcoholics or chronic cigarette smokers." Although Gallo often had his differences with the CDC, one could say that, epidemiologically speaking, he was on the same page.

Gallo told D'Eramo, "I would advocate sexual abstinence until this problem is solved. It may be a while, it may be a lifetime. I'm sorry, I'm doing my best." About transmission Gallo said, "I think it's close contact of any kind, like sharing a household, that may expose you to the virus."

At the time, Gallo was clearly the source of the government's public face of optimism about a possible vaccine. He said, "I'm not pessimistic about preventing disease. We will have a vaccine ready in a few years."

D'Eramo told Gallo, "Many gay men are afraid that people like Jerry Falwell and others of right-wing persuasion will use the HTLV-III tests results to recommend quarantine, or job restrictions, or even concentration camps. They're also concerned that all their names and addresses might be kept for a 'big round-up' someday." Gallo told D'Eramo, "If I believed that were going to happen to me, I would still be willing to take the chance, to take the gamble. I don't think Jerry Falwell has that kind of power, and although I would never recommend that somebody be quarantined, it is not irrational. They quarantined people for things in the past. But we're not going to spread HTLV-III through casual contact with people on the streets. That's clear from all the epidemiological data so far. But among our own friends, we need somebody to say that if we're not careful, we may all be dead. And maybe we all have to be super strong and super-sacrificing for a while and support the scientists who are trying to resolve this."

While Gallo was riding high on the credit of discovering the so-called cause of AIDS, throughout the rest of 1984 Teas continued to seek help in testing her ASFV hypothesis. She traveled to Italy, Spain, and England to meet with members of various members of their respective health ministries. Scientists in Italy were afraid to investigate a pig virus with which they had no experience. When she sought the help of the U.N.'s Food and Agriculture Organization, she was told that they would only investigate "unexplained illness among people if it occurred coincidently with an epidemic of ASFV." In an article she wrote for the *Native* she noted, "When I pointed out that this had indeed happened in Zaire, Haiti and the Cameroons, I was told that the Minister of Health [of those countries] would have to make the request for testing." Given the politics of ASFV that we had previously seen, *that* was not likely to happen.

Teas was successful in getting the Spanish Health Ministry to agree on further ASFV testing. Spain had had a problem with African swine fever in its pigs that year. She also visited the Pirbright Animal Research Center in England and was told that scientists would be willing to test her hypothesis if she would provide them with sera from AIDS patients. She returned to the United States and arranged to obtain AIDS sera from Dr. Michael Lange, an AIDS researcher in Manhattan. Early that summer of 1984, James D'Eramo and I nervously took a box containing fifty samples of blood from AIDS patients by taxi to LaGuardia Airport where we met Jane before she flew to London. She left the blood at Pirbright and then flew on to Nepal where she had a temporary job. Several months later she wrote a piece for the *Native* about her Pirbright experience: "In October, somewhat disappointed that I had not heard from anyone about the AIDS testing, I returned to England. They had not done the tests. I delicately indicated that I planned to remain in England until the tests were conducted and [subsequently] was surprised to learn that some of the sera had shown definitely positive results to African swine fever virus."

The scientist who performed the ASFV tests on the AIDS blood was Dr. Robert Downing. Downing had used virus from epidemics that had occurred in three different countries. Teas wrote in the *Native*, "It was particularly interesting that the 50 samples tested against ASFV [strains] from Zaire, the Cameroons, and Haiti were only positive for Haitian ASFV. This series of tests used the whole virus, whereas previous tests by Belgians and Haitians had used only a single viral protein. I was told there was nothing further I could do, and that they would certainly repeat the tests in the near future."

Teas flew back to New York and we were amazed when we saw the results. We looked forward to her writing up the results and submitting them to a scientific journal. But in order to do that she needed the cooperation of Dr. Downing. Unfortunately Downing subsequently refused to take any of Jane Teas's phone calls. And a woman who helped Teas set up the experiments also refused to respond to her inquiries. It was very strange. We were just beginning to get a sense of what we were dealing with.

1985: Throwing Down the Gauntlet

Because the *Native* was having financial problems, I was not able to keep D'Eramo on the payroll and he left the paper at the end of 1984. At the time I thought that a book written by Ann Giudici Fettner, *The Truth About AIDS*, was one of the best books on the subject, so I asked her to write periodically about the epidemic. In early 1985, she penned a piece for us on a disturbing epidemic of Multiple Sclerosis in Key West, Florida.

Fettner wrote, "Multiple Sclerosis (MS) is a mysterious illness which affects about 25,000 Americans. The disease gradually and irreversibly destroys the myelin of nerves, causing paralysis and death. Apparently an autoimmune phenomenon, MS sets the macrophage cells in action to literally eat away at the infected person's nerve tissues. . . . In Key West, at least 30 people are suffering from MS. Eight of them are nurses, who live and work in local hospitals. When the outbreak was first noted, there was speculation that it had some correlation with AIDS, but only one of the 30 is positive for LAV/HTLV-III. . . . Dr. Robert Gallo's group and the National Cancer Institute subsequently became involved, and they, with others, found that 60 percent of the MS patients have antibodies that react with proteins from HTLV. This may well be an artifact of autoimmunity, as the antibody seems to come and go in the patients. Because of the clustering of these unusual cases in Florida, close, prolonged contact—at least in the nurses—appears to be a factor in transmission, if a virus triggers the disease. . . . Researchers are trekking to the island community to try to solve the current mystery and find the cause of the disease."

Based on the fact that southern Florida was a major locus of AIDS and the fact that macrophages, which are a prime target of African swine fever virus, were involved, I wondered if the nurses were infected with ASFV. During that period I spoke with a clinician and researcher named Dr. Mark Whiteside who was working in Belle Glade, Florida. Whiteside felt that the presence of a retrovirus in AIDS patients was opportunistic and he told me that he suspected that government scientists had declared the wrong virus to be the cause of AIDS, that LAV (or HTLV-III) was actually a red herring. Whiteside suspected that AIDS was probably caused by an arbovirus which is usually an RNA virus that is characterized by its ability to be transmitted by insects. Whiteside urged the government to test AIDS patients for all known arboviruses. African swine fever virus, even though it is a DNA virus, is also characterized as an arbovirus.

Throughout the early years of the epidemic, a gay man named James Monroe had been a kind of "Deep Throat" for me both at the New York City Health Department and then at the CDC where he eventually worked in the director's office. The stories he told me about what was going on inside those organizations helped shape my evolving understanding of the questionable politics and pseudo-science of what would turn out to be an epidemic of lies. Monroe told me one day on the phone that while he was working with the CDC in New York City he had observed a peculiar thing about how the CDC determined who was positive for the AIDS virus. He said that when the CDC was trying to decide what HTLV-III antibody level actually constituted a real infection, that is, the dividing line between a positive and a negative reading, if two men, one heterosexual and one gay had the same exact borderline reading, the heterosexual's blood would be marked negative, and the gay's positive. It bothered Monroe and it more than bothered me. When Monroe began to express doubts about HTLV-III, he was transferred out of AIDS research and it was suggested by his superiors that he was suffering from "delusional thinking." He told me that the insinuation was that he was suffering from such thinking because he was gay and might himself be suffering from the effects of the virus which was capable of infecting the brain. (It was a kind of medicalized demonization that came to be a regular feature of dissent-bashing in the epidemic.) Oddly enough, after Monroe was transferred to a position in the CDC director's office, he told me that whenever his boss, James Mason, a devout Mormon, went to Washington, he spent a great deal of time with Orin Hatch, the anti-gay Mormon right-winger. Years later Monroe also informed me that all CDC decisions about AIDS were actually being made in the Reagan White House.

As time went on, I noticed that my phone conversations with the CDC's top AIDS researcher, James Curran, became increasingly strained as I began to ask more and more skeptical questions about the so-called AIDS retrovirus. Curran adopted a somewhat mocking and sarcastic style when talking to me. He once asked in an insulting, snark-inflected tone of voice whether I thought he was being "homo-phobic." One could say I was beginning to peer beneath one of the civil masks of the raw heterosexism that was actually the driving force of the CDC's epidemiology. Eventually he stopped returning my calls. It was now abundantly clear that the little gay newspaper in New York City would no longer be the CDC's stenographer. And we were going to pay a stiff price for that.

In late May of 1985, I attended a gay press awards ceremony and ran into Dr. Joseph Sonnabend, a gay Manhattan clinician who had a large AIDS practice and a great deal of insight into the questionable politics of AIDS research. He had been involved in interferon research and he was an outspoken critic of the idea that only one virus was the cause of AIDS. I was grateful to be able to call him on a regular basis with technical scientific questions about the epidemic, viruses and the immune system. At the press ceremony Sonnabend handed me a little gift that would change my life. It was a book, *Betrayers of the Truth: Fraud and Deceit in the Halls of Science,* which was written by *New York Times* science reporters Nicholas Wade and William Broad.

Sonnabend had grown increasingly indignant about the way Robert Gallo was claiming that he, and not the French scientists, had discovered the so-called cause of AIDS. To Sonnabend it seemed at the time like a double absurdity. HTLV-III wasn't really the cause *and* Gallo hadn't even really discovered it. Sonnabend was also convinced that a couple of Gallo's other discoveries—on which his reputation was based—had also been lifted from the work of other scientists.

I spent the weekend devouring the Wade and Broad book. By the time I finished it, scales had fallen from my eyes and I saw American science in a whole new light. The book made it clear that scientists could easily cover up each other's frauds if they were powerful enough. The book made the case that scientists basically did not like to expose other scientists' misdeeds *and they distrusted any form of outside scrutiny.* It was just as full of old-boy networks and protection rackets as the business world. The scientific world, as depicted by *Betrayers of the Truth,* was one in which scientists could easily get away with theft and fraud. Suddenly the idea that we could depend on the scientific process to expose any wrongdoing, or incorrect conclusions of a Robert Gallo, seemed pathetically naïve. The book, and my growing indignation about stories that had been emerging about Gallo's strange "scientific" behavior, inspired me to take the biggest risk of my publishing career. I decided to cross the Rubicon.

When I arrived at the office on Monday, I told Bruce Eves, the art director of *New York Native,* what I wanted on the cover of the forthcoming issue (June 3, 1985). Under a headline of "AIDSGATE BEGINS," I wanted, in the largest possible type, "SHOULD GALLO AND ESSEX BE IN JAIL?"

I then began working on a full page editorial and started putting together a news page of four stories to back up the cover. One was about a letter by Dr. A. Karpas of the Department of Haemotological Medicine at the University of Cambridge to the British publication *New Scientist*. Karpas's letter essentially challenged Gallo's claims that *he* had discovered HTLV-III. The Karpas letter outlined the chronology of Gallo's work and the Montagnier group's work, concluding that Gallo had conveniently discovered his retrovirus at the exact same time that he had succeeded in growing the retrovirus which the French had supplied to him.

I also wrote a brief story which pointed out that *New York Native* was not the first publication to challenge Gallo: "In the February 7, 1985, issue of . . . *New Scientist*, Omar Sattaur explained how Gallo's misclassification may have resulted in the false claim that he discovered the 'AIDS virus.' " Sattaur had stated, "Evidence is now mounting that Robert C. Gallo has misclassified the virus that causes AIDS. The result of this misclassification is that the world has ignored the true discoverers, Luc Montagnier and colleagues at the Institute Pasteur in Paris, and has given Gallo the credit instead."

Sattaur also wrote, "Gallo, head of the Laboratory of Tumor Cell Biology at the National Cancer Institute in Bethesda, Maryland, was convinced from the outset, and still is convinced, that the AIDS virus belongs to a family of viruses called HTLV, which he discovered in 1980. But there is new scientific evidence to prove he's wrong. HTLV stands for human T-cell leukemia virus. Two members of the group cause a type of cancer. The two viruses make T-cells multiply, in an uncontrolled manner. The AIDS virus, however, actually kills T-cells; yet Gallo calls the AIDS virus HTLV-III. While large sums of research time and money are spent on trying to understand how the AIDS virus fits into the HTLV group, thousands continue to die from AIDS." The same article reported that Montagnier was experiencing a lot of pressure to change the name of his virus from LAV to HTLV-III, but he refused to do so.

We also reported in *New York Native*, that in a speech before a group of medical writers in New York, in February 1985, Montagnier "was trying to tell them that there was something suspicious about the fact that the isolate of HTLV-III which Dr. Gallo 'discovered' was nearly identical to the isolate of LAV Montagnier and his team had identified months earlier at the Pasteur Institute."

I also added a disturbing story about Gallo which I had found in *Betrayers of the Truth*. I sensed that it might be a clue to Gallo's character. It was headlined "Gallo Was Witness to Scandal in 1981." The text follows:

> Robert C. Gallo was a witness to a major scandal involving scientific fraud in 1981, according to a book called *Betrayers of the Truth: Fraud and Deceit in the Halls of Science* by *New York Times* writers William Broad and Nicholas Wade (Touchstone/Simon and Shuster, 1982). Although Gallo was not implicated in the incidence of scientific fraud, the authors use him as an example of how scientists often do not blow the whistle on their colleagues when the inability to replicate their experiments makes them suspicious.
>
> The fraud was uncovered when a number of scientists were unable to replicate the work of Cornell University cancer researcher Mark Spector. According to Broad and Wade, Spector was a brilliant young researcher whom many expected eventually to win a Nobel Prize. Many of the world's leading cancer researchers suspected something was wrong in Spector's experiment with the products of tumor-causing genes, but no one stepped forward to ask if fraudulent procedures were involved. One scientist explained that Spector's work was so "beautiful and convincing" the scientist was "seduced" into working with Spector. When other scientists couldn't repeat Spector's experiments, they merely gave up and didn't publicly challenge his credibility.
>
> Gradually, scientists began to notice that Spector's experiments "only worked when he was around to do them" until one of his colleagues realized there was "forgery" involved. The results of the experiments had appeared in the "prestigious" magazine *Science*. According to Broad and Wade it was eventually discovered that Spector "possessed neither an M.A. nor a B.A. from the University of Cincinnati as he had

claimed."

"Why wasn't the falsity of Spector's result discovered much earlier?" Wade and Broad ask in their book. "Why did none of the many biologists caught up in his theory not try first to replicate some of the basic results? The answer is: they did. Their failure to get the same answers as Spector should have stopped the theory dead in its tracks. It didn't."

And one of the scientists who found that he could not repeat Spector's experiments was Robert Gallo.

One of the main points the authors try to make in their book is that the notion of science as a "strictly logical process . . . rigorously checked by peer scrutiny and the replication of experiments" is largely a myth. A sick joke. According to the authors, scientists who are unable to replicate others' experiments are more likely either to assume they are performing the experiment incorrectly, or to quit the project in which they are involved.

On the news page, we included the response from the National Cancer Institute to our request for an interview with Gallo: "Robert Gallo would not return the *Native*'s phone calls, nor did he issue a statement about the allegations that his work on HTLV-III constitutes scientific fraud. A spokesperson for the National Cancer Institute told the *Native*, 'The charges are preposterous, and we will comment no further.'"

Below is my full page editorial from that issue titled "AIDSGATE":

It's time every scientist in the world with a shred of integrity began asking whether certain members of their community are up to their necks in scientific fraud.

There are at least two allegations that must be resolved immediately before public health guidelines for any treatment or diagnostic test based on the work of Dr. Robert Gallo of the National Cancer Institute, Dr. Max Essex of the Harvard School of Public Health, and their colleagues can be trusted by the American public and their physicians. The fact that these allegations are being whispered privately among scientists is a disgrace to the reputation of American science.

Tragically, cowardice abounds among many who have shown great courage in the past. Major scientific and medical publications have actually published articles which may have contained falsified test results and other scientific fraud.

Allegation #1

That Robert Gallo "discovered" the virus Dr. Luc Montagnier of the Pasteur Institute gave to him—i.e. that Gallo's lab "stole" the discovery from the French, after ignoring the French discovery for over a year, thereby setting treatment and vaccine research back immeasurably.

The issue of "virus lifting" might seem academic and irrelevant to uninformed Americans, but certainly it has implication for the ethics and validity of American AIDS research right now. If Gallo is the kind of man who would ignore others' significant breakthroughs and then falsely claim to have made the same discovery himself—and get away with it—what else would he be willing—and able—to falsify, and for whose convenience? What small, seemingly insignificant matters about the so-called AIDS virus might he also be fudging on—or overlooking completely? Do we have a virus-lifter running AIDS research at the National Cancer Institute?

We've been told that Gallo has had lunch dates at the White House. Who is Gallo's boss, anyway? Is AIDS policy being set in the Reagan Administration by open homophobes such as Patrick Buchanan?

Allegation #2

That the linking of an AIDS associated virus with HTLV-I and HTLV-II was a deliberate attempt to confuse scientists and the public, to enjoy acclaim, and to obtain grants and other benefits, including public monies. Such a deliberate linkage would constitute scientific fraud—and not one word of it can be tolerated during an emergency that many predict will affect every human life on the planet. Are we really supposed to believe that, after all his experience with HTLV-I and HTLV-II, Gallo could innocently have made such a mistake?

Sleaze Factor #1

Why has no one in the medical press decried Gallo's control of "his" virus. You'd think he was the sole possessor of the Coca Cola formula (albeit, in this case possibly stolen), the way other scientists have accepted and sustained his monopoly. The *Native* pointed this out last December.

Perhaps the most circumstantially convincing evidence that the powers that be are "protecting" something are the regulations Dr. Robert Gallo of the National Institutes of Health has imposed on "his" virus, HTLV-III. First, a higher level of security clearance is now required, eliminating many scientists. Secondly, only those people to whom Gallo personally gives the virus may work on it, and they may not give it to anyone else. Third, and most damning, only papers on which Gallo is a co-author may be published from work done on "his" virus. This means that any evidence contrary to the HTLV-III theory would remain unpublished.

Sleaze Factor #2

Gallo's Media Fan Club

Not only has Gallo found a way to control the flow of medical information about "his" virus, he has also bamboozled members of the lay media (we won't name them here; they know who they are) creating a coterie of groupies who have been given the privilege of calling the esteemed scientist "Bob."

We remember all too well the day we discussed AIDS with a *Wall Street Journal* reporter. With more than a hint of satisfaction in her voice, she let drop the fact that she had "talked to Bob Gallo the other day."

The formation of this "Bob Club" among reporters is at least part of the reason the real story about AIDS is not getting out. Too many media "Moonies" are giving "Bob" a free ride.

The "Bob Club" should disband, and these reporters should start doing their job—instead of believing everything "Bob" tells them.

Essex Allegation

Dr. Max Essex of the Harvard School of Public Health has the responsibility of making sure that his students conduct sound scientific research. His own research should also be sound (if only to set a good example), and should be absent of any form of fraud or falsification.

Essex has been a longtime collaborator with Gallo. In good conscience, how has Essex been able to remain silent?

Why this is important

Why are these allegations so important, and why must they be resolved immediately? Because the crucial decisions we make about our own health, and the decisions our doctors make, are life-and-death decisions—they cannot be based on fraudulent science. We cannot tolerate inertia on the part of scientists and public health administrators who feel they can look the other way while other scientists steal viruses and push them into phony categories.

We've been smelling a rat in AIDS research, and the odor is now overpowering. Indeed, AIDS has become AIDSGATE.

After Gallo saw that issue of *New York Native*, I received an unexpected phone call from him. It inspired another intense issue of the paper (June 17, 1985) and another long editorial, titled "Castro and the Two Gallos":

On Friday, May 31, Dr. Robert C. Gallo of the National Cancer Institute was scheduled to appear at a West Coast conference held by the Association for the Advancement of Science. He was also supposed to be interviewed by National Public Radio for their program, *All Things Considered*. The program's producers wanted Gallo to respond to my recent allegations, which include the charge that his "discovery" of HTLV-III was in fact nothing more than the rediscovery of another research team's identical virus.

I've followed Gallo's behavior for a couple of years now. He has emerged as the most powerful and influential figure in American AIDS research, partly by dint of his personality. Gallo is famous for his lightning bolt appearances at scientific conferences; intimidating, sweeping performances that are really "press opportunities" for the media and his colleagues to photograph him. Perhaps because of this demeanor, the science of Robert Gallo as applied to AIDS has generally not been the sort other scientists could easily or readily challenge in public. I've also heard that scientific papers which contradict Gallo's "findings" are generally rejected by the leading medical journals. Such is the man's power.

I called Gallo's office on the morning of May 31, to find out whether he'd gone to Los Angeles as scheduled. Not surprisingly, his secretary told me he was in a meeting and asked, "Would he know what this is in reference to?" I replied that I thought he would. Within a half-hour, I was told that someone describing himself as "Mr. Ortleb's star witness" was waiting to speak to me on the phone.

It was Gallo.

I want here to present the salient points of our conversation (during which I did most of the listening), because I think Robert Gallo has had more impact on the course of the AIDS epidemic than anyone in America. I also think he is deeply disturbed.

I began the conversation by asking what must have struck Gallo as an odd question. Had he told Loretta McLaughlin, medical writer for the *Boston Globe*, that he didn't know anything about African swine fever virus (as McLaughlin had reported to me)? He replied that the only thing he knew about the virus was that I was interested in it. He then told me in rapid succession:

1. I had made a tremendous mistake, the mistake of my lifetime (in accusing him of fraud.)

2. He "couldn't be mad at me" because I "was sincere."

3. There was something very "big and wrong with my thinking."

4. I was either being "manipulated by a schizophrenic scientist" (he would not tell me the name of the scientist), or I was "irrational."

5. I should "try to be a friend."

6. I could be compared to President Reagan, because I "make statements with no basis in fact."

7. Margaret Heckler "perhaps had not done the right thing" at her historic press conference called to announce Gallo's findings a year ago.

8. He didn't need HTLV-III to be considered a success; he had been warned to stay away from AIDS because "situations like this" (I presume he meant the *Native*'s AIDSGATE allegations) might arise. "I don't *need* AIDS," he said.

9. He didn't know how to do the right thing with the press; he had never called a press conference in his life; he was a nervous wreck at the Heckler press conference; he had told Heckler that he felt he had enough data and that he felt he knew the etiology of the disease. He blamed his erratic performance at another press conference on the fact that his father had just died. He told me that his father had worked his way from welder to businessman. He pointed out that he doesn't like publicity. "I do not want to be noticed," he said.

10. He felt that he had the idea and the methodology that led to the discovery of LAV and that, in science, ideas and methodology are everything. I told him that providing methodology didn't mean he could lay claim to every discovery associated with his methodology. (I didn't say it then, but I'll say it now: By that logic, HTLV-III was discovered by Leeuwenhoek, inventor of the microscope.")

11. He said that Omar Sattaur, who wrote a piece criticizing Gallo in *New Scientist*, "didn't know the difference between a bacterium and a virus."

12. He wouldn't dignify A. Karpas (of Cambridge University) with a response to his letter to *New Scientist* (3/28/85) suggesting that there was something fishy about the fact that Gallo's lab discovered HTLV-III just three months after they had been able to grow LAV, the virus the Pasteur Institute had already associated with AIDS.

13. The nomenclature of HTLV-III was decided in an agreement with Japanese researchers in Cold Spring Harbor.

14. He didn't want the virus he named HTLV-III to be called "the AIDS virus," because it would stigmatize homosexuals. (I love the idea of taxonomy by charity.) He also said, "I don't care what the virus is called."

15. When I told him that I called one of his ex-employees who said Gallo was not really responsible for the work done on HTLV-I and Interleukin-II (other Gallo "discoveries" which might result in a fraudulently gained Nobel Prize), he said that he had two disgruntled ex-lab workers who had gone nowhere in science. (When I asked him for their names, he wouldn't tell me.)

16. He said that there were competitive scientists who were out to "cut" his "legs off."

17. I told Gallo a few of the basics about African swine fever virus, and he thanked me. He seemed to know nothing about the virus.

18. I asked him if he would be livid if one of his colleagues thought that AIDS was caused by some agent other than HTLV-III and failed to share their knowledge with Gallo. He said he would be "doubly livid."

19. I reminded Gallo that he had discussed African swine fever virus with James D'Eramo, Ph.D., in the now famous interview the *Native* published last summer. D'Eramo: "Do you think other viruses, like CMV or EBV play a role in development of AIDS? Dr. Jane Teas told us a long time ago about the idea of African swine fever virus coming from Africa to Haiti

and then from Haiti to America." Gallo: "It turns out that even though she had the wrong virus, she seems to have the right idea about the origins of the virus. She didn't have any knowledge of HTLV-III; she didn't know it existed—why should she?—so hers was a good insight. I agree." Gallo called this a "miscommunication" on D'Eramo's part. (The interview was tape recorded in full.)

20. Gallo continually told me, "If you'd only read the science, if you only understood the science." I told him I wouldn't be browbeaten by him or his so-called science, even if most of the AIDS researchers in America are afraid of him. I told him that if he wanted to learn more about swine fever, he should call Dr. William Hess of the U.S. Department of Agriculture's Plum Island facility, or ask his collaborator at the Harvard School of Public health, Dr. Max Essex. He said, "I will look into it."

21. I told him that scientists who didn't believe that HTLV-III is the cause of AIDS can't get funding if they don't write his virus into their grant requests. He said he had nothing to do with funding, and that he agreed it was wrong to censor grant requests on that basis. He alleged that he had not gotten one additional cent of funding as a result of his discovery.

22. At one point in the conversation, Gallo listed his achievements with HTLV-III. He was proud that they had proved that HTLV-III doesn't cause Kaposi's sarcoma, that the virus replicates in the brain, that his lab was the first to sequence the virus, and that they were the first to link it with thrombocytopenia.

23. He told me that the original papers on LAV written by the French researchers would never have been published if he had not intervened. He argued that the French did not link the virus to the disease.

24. I asked if he had been reading the AIDS coverage in the *Native*. He said that he had not. I urged him to read the *Native*. He remarked that this would require some bravery on his part. (It would.)

Our conversation left me with the impression of a

man who is to say the least, emotionally very high strung. His claims of powerlessness are contradicted by the former associate who told me that Gallo had very little to do with the discovery of HTLV-I and Interleukin-II. The associate did not want his name used because, he said, Gallo could destroy his career. He told me that Gallo's ex-employees are "a gold mine of information about Gallo" and that I "would not believe some of the things that go on in his lab."

Earlier that very morning, Gallo had called Ann Giudici Fettner, co-author of *The Truth about AIDS* (which recently won the American Medical Writers Association Award) and a frequent contributor to the *Native*. During the conversation, he told Fettner that, because of her association with us, she would never be able to write about science again, because no one at the National Institutes of Health would talk to her. Fettner remains undaunted. To say the least, she cannot be bullied.

Then, on the morning of June 4, Gallo called Dr. Hess at Plum Island. According to Hess, Gallo asked him "how the whole African Swine disease thing got started," and who Jane Teas was. (Gallo has a slight memory problem.) Hess told me he found it rather difficult to believe that Gallo was so ignorant about swine fever. He described Gallo's speaking manner as "hyper," and said that Gallo was "ranting and raving."

Hess is a rather circumspect, soft-spoken, highly methodical man. He said that Gallo fired questions at him so rapidly, he hardly had time to respond. Gallo asked Hess whether African swine fever virus killed T-cells, and as Hess was about to answer, Gallo snapped, "Well, I guess you don't have the information there." Hess said that Gallo kept going on and on about his "115 isolates of HTLV-III," and eventually offered to send one of them to Hess. (Hess is not interested in Gallo's isolates.)

Gallo began to harangue Hess, insisting that he has nothing to do with funding, even though that's of no interest to Hess, whose work is primarily focused on trying to understand the nature of African swine fever virus, the basis of Hess's reputation and career.

By this point, the call apparently turned from an inquiry about swine fever into another defense brief from the "star witness." Hess told me that he couldn't quite ascertain what the purpose of Gallo's call was, and that he was getting tired of receiving calls from researchers who seemed bent on "finding out how much I know" about the possible connection be-tween AIDS and African swine fever virus.

Hess didn't know where Gallo was calling him from, but it must have been Boston, because on that same day, June 4, Gallo made a presentation to medical researchers at Boston University.

Gallo's presentation, according to a source who wishes to remain anonymous, contained interesting scientific observations as well as a rather bizarre slide projection intended to explain how Gallo's virus, HTLV-III, destroys lymphocytes. Uninfected lymphocytes were illustrated on the slides as little "happy faces." Infected lymphocytes were drawn as bald women trying to seduce the happy faces. Once seduced, the little happy faces died and became angels, who went to lymphocyte heaven. (*Native* readers may be on the floor laughing at this point, but reportedly most scientists present did not say anything, although there were apparently some groans in the audience. One scientist who was present told us, "I found myself trying to deny that he was actually portraying it in that manner.")

After the conference, Gallo went out to eat with some of his colleagues. The anonymous source told us that, at the lunch, Gallo told his companions that he blamed Fidel Castro for sending "diseased homosexuals" to America during the Mariella boat lift, thus bringing AIDS into the U.S. Gallo made extremely negative remarks about Haiti, and referred to homosexuals as "homos." According to our source, "He went into a whole thing about people fucking sheep; he was berserk on the topic."

Gallo had just told the audience at the conference that 65% of the blood donors in Brazil were testing positive for HTLV-III, and expressed surprise that there were so many homosexuals in Brazil. (The way he reportedly put it was that he "didn't realize there were so many of 'them' in Brazil.") Our source said that throughout the conference and the luncheon Gallo gave the impression of being a man who is deeply "erotophobic and homophobic." One of the top medical writers in America, with whom I shared this report, concurred, saying, "It sounds like Gallo is losing his grip on reality."

To borrow some of Gallo's own "scientific language," I think we have discovered two isolates: Gallo-I and Gallo-II (there may be more to come.)

Gallo-I is a reasonable scientist, who knows a great deal about retroviruses (though not a thing about African swine fever virus). Gallo-I is a well-respected scientist, whose name appears on a lot of scientific papers for work he may have, at times, done himself. Gallo-I is a jet-setting, fast-talking retro-virologist who craves the approval of the scientific community, an award-winning scientist awaiting the preordained day he will be called to Stockholm to receive that ultimate honor, the Nobel Prize.

Gallo-II is a fraudulent, vindictive, arrogant, anti-gay little bully. Gallo-II makes sure that anyone who disagrees with him suffers bad consequences professionally. Gallo-II is xenophobic and racist. Gallo-II is obsessed with the idea that AIDS is caused by people sleeping with sheep and green monkeys (hopefully not in threesomes).

Fools like Dr. James Mason, Director of the Centers for Disease Control, who recently told a group of people with AIDS that Gallo "had his problems, but he's a brilliant scientist," may subscribe to the notion that we have to live with Gallo-I and Gallo-II

I don't.

Gallo told me that he thought a schizophrenic scientist was manipulating me. If any schizophrenic scientist has tried to manipulate the entire scientific establishment, it is Dr. Robert C. Gallo himself.

In the same issue of the *Native*, I wrote a short ominous news story (that captured the menacing atmosphere of the epidemic) headlined "Reagan Administration Considering AIDS Quarantine: CDC Director Reveals Discussions to PWAs." It began, "At a May 20 meeting in Washington, between a group representing people with AIDS in America and Dr. James Mason, the director of the Centers for Disease Control revealed that the Reagan Administration is considering a quarantine of people with AIDS. Paul Boneberg who heads the Mobilization Against AIDS, told the *Native* that Mason revealed to the stunned group of 12 people that he had been at an administration meeting that morning at which quarantine for AIDS patients had been discussed. According to Boneberg, Mason says he is personally against quarantine. The group pleaded with Mason to provide more money for public education on AIDS, to which Mason responded, 'Do you really believe gay men can be changed through education?' The head of the CDC is from a Mormon college in Utah which allegedly has used electroshock 'aversion therapy' to 'change' homosexuals. Boneberg told the *Native* that his impression was that Mason is totally unapologetic for the administration's approach to the AIDS crisis. He said he was shocked at how insensitive Mason was to the PWAs in his presence . . . . Boneberg feels that the meeting with Mason was unproductive and that dialogue with the Reagan Administration has reached a dead end."

On June 14, 1985, I visited Albany at the invitation of Mel Rosen, the director of New York State's AIDS Institute. There I met with Andrew Fleck, an advisor to the State Health Commissioner David Axelrod. I had talked with Fleck several times on the phone during the preceding year and he had seemed to be a sophisticated theoretician on matters of epidemiology and public health.

Fleck was an aristocratic-looking registered Republican in a Democratic state administration. I wrote in the *Native*, "His standards of excellence in epidemiology put the Centers for Disease Control to shame, and I had told him on more than one occasion that the AIDS epidemic could use some of his experience and wisdom. But he has maintained that he prefers to work outside of the limelight. I trust that he's part of the reason State Health Commissioner David Axlerod has not become a proponent of the fuzzy CDC epidemiological data or the virological fraud coming out of the National Cancer Institute. Fleck seems to play the role of the avuncular professional wall off of which [Axlerod] can bounce ideas before taking action."

Joining us was Dr. Jean Dodds, a prominent scientist in the New York State Health Department who had been the chief of the state's Hematology Laboratory for two years. I had called her on and off during the previous year-and-a-half, trying to enlist her in Teas's efforts to test the ASFV AIDS hypothesis. But she wouldn't have any of it. I had assumed that she didn't know anything about African swine fever virus; certainly she'd never let on that she did.

When Rosen and I arrived in Albany around lunchtime, we went directly to Fleck's office. Dodds was there. She was a single, rather perky, fortyish woman who talked rapidly and was capable of leaping deftly from issue to issue. I wrote, in the *Native*, that she was "brainy and always seemed to have ideas moving on the forecourt and back-court."

I was quite surprised when, upon our arrival at Fleck's office, she handed me three research papers on African swine fever virus which had been published in the *American Journal of Veterinary Medicine* and in *Veterinary Pathology*. The lead author on these papers, J. F. Edwards, was someone I had actually talked to a year or so before that. I had tracked him down at a university in Texas to question him about the relationship between African swine fever and AIDS. On the phone he had been very hostile about such a suggestion. Edwards angrily insisted that there was absolutely no similarity between AIDS and African swine fever. When I pointed out that pigs with ASFV developed pneumonia just like AIDS patients, he retorted that the pneumonia in pigs was more like tuberculosis than the Pneumocystis carinii pneumonia that was occurring in AIDS. (It became clear, as the AIDS epidemic progressed, that tuberculosis was in fact a major problem in AIDS.) Edwards's research interest at the time was thrombocytopenia in swine fever. (Thrombocytopenia is basically a disorder in which the blood fails to coagulate properly.) From my own research I knew that thrombocytopenia was a problem in AIDS but Edwards seemed annoyed when I pointed out that AIDS and ASFV had that pathology in common. My conversation with him *was* another puzzling moment in the AIDS era when I ran into an uncanny hostility that seemed to be coming out of nowhere. AIDS had the whole country on edge, but I now think it was more than that.

That day in Albany, when I told Jean Dodds that I had spoken to Edwards, she said that she had been one of his students which surprised me.

Fleck took us to lunch and when Fleck ordered veal, I followed suit. Dodds glared at us. She pointed out that she was an animal rights activist and she asked if we were really going to order veal. She went on to describe the horrible things that meat companies do to calves. She obviously wanted us to change our orders, but Fleck shrugged her off and stuck to his veal. I felt awkward at first, but I grew annoyed. Dodds then told us that she had been up late the night before because she had to put one of her "hemophiliacs to sleep." She lived with several hemophiliac German Shepherds in a farm-house in Albany.

The conversation at lunch was basically about Gallo and African swine fever virus. Fleck described Gallo as "a burden to science," but tended to speak of him in a kindlier manner than I have. We also discussed a member of the Centers for Disease Control, Richard Rothenberg, who was stationed in the New York State Health Department. I complained to Fleck and Dodds about the CDC's ability to impose its own agendas on state and local governments by providing them with staff and money. The CDC had very long arms.

Over our controversial veal and her pasta, we discussed what the State of New York could do to test the hypothesis that AIDS and African swine fever were related. Fleck said that when Teas had introduced the hypothesis two years earlier, it had made a great deal of sense to him, considering the geographic distribution of the two epidemics. I told them that I was planning on writing an editorial attacking Gallo for placing "T-cell blinders" on the scientific community that recognizing the full scope of what AIDS was. I also told them that Kaposi's sarcoma was probably one of the most visible clues that AIDS was a form of African swine fever. Dodds bristled at the notion that lesions in pigs with ASFV might be at all similar to Kaposi's sarcoma lesions. She made a few arcane remarks about necrosis of the endothelial cells in African swine fever virus infected pig tissue being a totally different phenomenon in KS. I told Dodds that she was talking about the acute cases of ASFV infection as opposed to infection with the chronic strains, which Teas has suspected might behind the AIDS epidemic. She let me know, rather cuttingly, that she knew the difference. I was caught off guard, surprised that Dodds knew so much about ASFV. I had brought along 30 research papers on ASFV and had planned to discuss them with her, but we never got to them.

Dodds didn't see the epidemiological patterns of ASFV as being either convincing or interesting. She said that everything I had told her about swine fever and AIDS could be said about parvovirus and AIDS, an area of research interest for her. I responded by saying that if she thought that AIDS is caused by parvovirus, she was in an excellent position to get *her* idea tested. She agreed that every idea should be tested which made her sound open-minded, but I suspected it was just another way of saying ASFV was another crazy dime-a-dozen idea about the cause of AIDS.

Mel Rosen was getting a little impatient as the lunch ended. He had told me in the weeks before that he didn't like the idea that the testing on African swine fever had been basically stonewalled at every turn for two years. While he insisted that he had no investment in swine fever as the cause, he continually told me, "I just want to do the right thing." He turned to Dodds and Fleck and said, "What can we do for Ortleb?"

Dodds said that she would be overseeing the grants process of New York State's AIDS Institute, and she suggested that I ask Teas to apply for a New York State research grant.

I wasn't pleased. I thought that just meant more delays, more foot-dragging. I told Dodds that the problem wasn't money but rather getting the cooperation of the U.S. Department of Agriculture. The USDA's assistance was required to do any research on African swine fever virus.

Fleck and Dodds assured me that if a researcher got a state grant and then had trouble getting African swine fever virus for testing purposes from the USDA, the state would step in. I replied, "Why don't you step in now, Jean? Why don't you try to test sera from ten people with AIDS for the presence of African swine fever virus?"

She responded, "I can't drop everything and just test your hypothesis."

I said, "I didn't ask you to *drop everything* and test the hypothesis."

It was getting a little unfriendly and Rosen looked exasperated. I felt like Dodds was playing games with me and that I was about to reach another dead end. Dodds got up to leave the table and I wondered why I even had bothered to come up to Albany. Rosen had made the prospects of something happening in Albany seem better than this.

Rosen took me back to his state office, where I was to wait for two hours until we both got the train back to Manhattan. While he attended a meeting, I sat down and started to read the three research papers on African swine fever virus that Dodds had given me. When I looked at the authors of the papers I got quite a shock. On all three of the ASFV papers Jean Dodds was listed as one of the researchers. Why hadn't she told me that she had personal research experience with the virus? Something didn't smell right. In order to do ASFV research she had to have had some kind of contact with the USDA at Plum Island. That she had co-authored one of the papers on thrombocytopenia in ASFV was disturbing to me because that was also a tell-tale sign of AIDS. If she knew so much about ASFV, why did she refuse to acknowledge their obvious similarities? I found it bizarre that she didn't discuss her own ASFV research at lunch. What was really going on?

When Rosen returned from his meeting, he took me to meet Richard Rothenberg, the CDC's man in Albany. Rothenberg was a tiny man who somewhat resembled Woody Allen. I had heard from Rosen that he was not respected by the top people at the state's health department. As I understood it, his job was to convince Albany to faithfully follow the CDC agenda, which I was gradually becoming convinced, was more about politics than real science. I had been told that in meeting after meeting Rothenberg had been trying to convince the skeptical health commissioner that HTLV-III was the real cause of AIDS.

Rosen left me alone in a room with Rothenberg. He asked me what I thought of Fleck. I told him I thought he was a brilliant scientist. He didn't seem to agree. I told Rothenberg that I had heard he was having problems with Axelrod. He told me that the problem was that there were a lot of "advocates" in the New York State Health Department. I gathered that he didn't see himself as any kind of "advocate." He went on to tell me that the problem with his boss was that he "shoots from the hip." We turned to the subject of African swine fever virus, and he asked me why I was an "advocate" of that theory. Although I resented the rather patronizing insinuations implicit in the term "advocate," I began to go over the list of reasons. I borrowed a piece of paper and drew a rough map that included Africa, Haiti, Cuba and Brazil. I drew an arrow point from Zaire to the Caribbean Basin. I said, "Let's see, swine fever seems to have gone from Zaire to the Dominican Republic in . . . ."

"In 1978," he said.

"Oh yes," I said, wondering how he knew. I continued, And then it seems to have shown up in Brazil . . . ."

"In 1978," he interrupted. He then said that he understood why I saw similarities, but that there were two important differences. The first, he said was that in swine fever there is a tremendous release of pyrogen (a substance released by macrophages that causes fever), and that in swine fever the central pathological event is vasculitis. (Unfortunately Rothenberg may have known more about African swine fever than AIDS. His two big differences turned out to be two big similarities.) Interestingly, Rothenberg did say that if African swine fever was the cause, it would eventually come out and said that if it did the role I was playing might make it come out sooner. Most surprisingly, he also told me that Don Francis, the CDC researcher who told us that the CDC's testing for ASFV in AIDS patients had come out negative, was now saying that ASFV might be a cofactor in AIDS. That didn't make any sense to me. I asked Rothenberg if Francis was being facetious and he replied that Francis was serious.

On the train back to Manhattan, I grilled Rosen on Dodds, asking if he thought Dodds was playing some kind of political game with the ASFV issue. "If Jean Dodds is a villain, I'll go nuts," Rosen said. I told him I found it odd that she was intimately involved in both AIDS and ASFV research. It was quite a coincidence.

The more I thought about the Albany meetings, the more annoyed I became. On the following Monday, I sent a Mailgram to State Health Commissioner David Axlerod: "It's amazing that Jean Dodds knows so much about African swine fever virus and has connections to Plum Island, USDA, and yet has done so little to make sure that men, women and children with AIDS are not actually infected with swine fever virus. This is a moral and scientific outrage. We raise this issue in the next "AIDSGATE" section of *New York Native*. Please tell Rich Rothenberg that there is vasculitis in AIDS. Rich should try to keep up with the AIDS literature instead of just trying to hoodwink you. . . . I suggest that we meet for a full discussion without the presence of Dodds as soon as possible."

Several days later, I received the following letter from Dodds:

June 19, 1985, 6:10 a.m.

> Dear Chuck,
>
> After we met last Friday, I had intended to drop you a personal note to say how much I enjoyed meeting

you and that I liked you a lot and found you very clever and intuitive. By the way, it's a beautiful clear morning as I sit at the dining room table and look through my many windows onto the hills in the distance. Country living is peaceful and comforting.

You can imagine my surprise and hurt feelings when I learned on Monday morning of your telegram to Commissioner Axelrod (whom I admire very much) and your concerns about me and my role in the African swine fever "issue." I had just returned from teaching our alternate site counselors and had proudly told them of our Friday meeting and joint decision to encourage other avenues of research on AIDS—including looking into the cofactor/role of ASF virus and trying to obtain reagents should an appropriately designed study plan be developed.

We invited you to Albany (in fact it was my urging along with Mel [Rosen's] encouragement that developed the invitation) in good faith and with honest intentions—because I feel scientifically and medically that anyone's or any theory has the right to be pursued. In fact, freedom of scientific inquiry is what science is all about. We are now embarrassed and feel somewhat betrayed by what happened. My dear friend (if you'll allow me to call you a friend), how can I or we help you to achieve your goal unless you trust us to stick to our agreement? Surely by being so zealous about the conspiracy you fear exists and then extending it to include the very group that has agreed to help you, you are potentially undermining the effort and creating a situation whereby despite what we do to promote a proper study of the matter, the department may not agree—for fear of being "slapped in the face" again! I'm really sorry about all this. Personally, I'm disappointed that you think ill of me or my intentions, but my conscience is absolutely clear. I've dedicated my life to public service and compassionate concern for all living things. I stand on my loyalty, sincerity, and honesty. I still want to help you and will do so in good faith. I've already contacted Plum Island as promised, and the department has assured access to the reagents needed should a study like the one we suggested be undertaken.

The ball is in your court. Hopefully, you can reach out to us (me) again as I'm doing in this letter.

God bless and care for you.

Shortly after that, the Health Commissioner of New York State ordered that blood from people with AIDS be tested for the presence of African swine fever virus. In the July 15 issue, I wrote an editorial that outlined some of my concerns about the predispositions and trustworthiness of the people who would be doing the blood testing:

> As we went to press with this issue, there were no available details about the nature of the intended state research which might end two years of speculation in this publication about why the government has avoided investigating the obvious connection between AIDS and African swine fever, the virtually identical disease in pigs. Concern about the tremendous economic impact of a swine fever outbreak may explain the Centers for Disease Control's avoidance of a serious investigation.
>
> In the February 22, 1984, issue of the *South Jersey Courier-Post*, Judy Petsonk wrote about Dr. James Curran, head of the CDC's AIDS Task Force, and his feelings about Jane Teas's theory that AIDS is caused by African swine fever virus: "Curran also said he was afraid that Teas's theory might make people afraid to eat pork, thus harming the pork industry in the U.S." If Curran has put the welfare of the pork industry before the welfare of patients, it would not be the first time the Centers for Disease Control put ethics on a back burner while patients suffered or died. James H. Jones's book, *Bad Blood: The Tuskegee Syphilis Experiment, A Tragedy of Race and Medicine* (Free Press, 1981), documents in full a case in which the Centers for Disease Control apparently found nothing wrong with continuing a 1930s experiment in which government doctors studied the effects of untreated syphilis in 400

black Alabama sharecroppers, who did not know they had the disease. The Tuskegee experiment has many interesting parallels with the way AIDS is being handled by the Public Health Service; the current paucity of funding for therapeutic research projects seems to be a deliberate strategy to let AIDS patients die.

Curran's attitude toward the potential victims of AIDS, as described by Robert Gallo of the National Cancer Institute, strongly resembles the attitudes of white doctors toward blacks in the late nineteenth century, also explored by Jones in his book. In our August 27, 1984, issue, Gallo told the *Native*, "I have heard that there are some who are so sexually driven that they are like alcoholics. . . . I have heard that from Dr. Curran. There are some that are so hypersexual that they're like alcoholics or chronic cigarette smokers." From *Bad Blood*: "White physicians of the late nineteenth and early twentieth centuries blamed the decline in black health on self-destructive be-havioral traits. . . . Physicians hammered away at the black man's distaste for honest labor, fondness for alcohol, proclivity to crime and sexual vices, disregard for personal hygiene, ignorance of the laws or good nutrition, and total indifference to his own health. [Black people] had only themselves to blame."

Whether such an attitude toward the gay community also pervades the New York State Health Department remains to be seen. Frances Tarlton, spokesperson for the department, seems preoccupied with the sexuality of those who suspect AIDS could be caused by African swine fever. She told *Newsday* (June 27, 1985), "The State Health Department will test a theory that African swine fever virus may be linked to AIDS, a belief held by few scientists but supported by some in the homosexual community."

One non-gay, non-journalist who has suspected a link between AIDS and swine fever is Dr. Frederick Maurer, a retired Lt. Colonel of the U.S. Army [and an experienced ASFV researcher]. On July 3, 1983,

Maurer wrote to the CDC about the connection, but was ignored by Curran.

A swine fever outbreak could cost $25 billion annually. It is reasonable to expect that there are people in the government who would find it more advantageous to cover up any presence of swine fever in the U.S., and to let the disease continue spreading among the pig (and/or human) population, rather than suffer the economic consequences that would follow an admission of swine fever is in the U.S. (One ASFV scientist informs us that Brazil has adopted such a policy.)

In a staff paper from the Institute of Agriculture, Forestry and Home Economics entitled "Potential Economic Consequences of African Swine Fever and Its Control in the United States," E.H. McCauley and W.B. Sundquist wrote, "It is clear that because of the large size of the U.S. swine production industry and the large volume of domestic consumption and export marketing of pork and related products, economic impacts of endemic African swine fever will quickly run into the billions of dollars." The writers argue, "In addition to the loss of exports for pork and related products should ASFV become endemic in the U.S., some countries, particularly those with domestic swine production of their own, are likely to place a partial or complete embargo on the imports of other agricultural products from the U.S. for fear that these products may serve as carriers of ASF to their swine populations. Though it is difficult to isolate and quantify the magnitude of such potential losses, U.S. agricultural exports, among which grains, soybeans, cotton, and animal products predominate, currently total to about $25 billion annually."

That report was published in 1979.

Ironically, the United States Department of Agriculture distributes many pamphlets to American pig farmers warning them to be vigilant and aware of African swine fever's symptoms. According to one such pamphlet, "Plans for a U.S. emergency eradication program against ASFV have already been developed. State and federal animal health authorities will begin eradication immediately upon confirmation of an outbreak." The same pamphlet warns, "If any hogs show signs of African swine fever or Hog Cholera, notify your veterinarian, state or federal animal health official, or your country agricultural agent at once."

There is already some evidence that swine fever is in the country and is being ignored by federal health officials. Dr. Peter Drotman of the Centers for Disease Control told Joe Nicholson of the *New York Post* six months ago, "Federal doctors stopped investigation of the pig disease even though its only study found that 'a few' AIDS patients tested positive for the pig virus."

If it does turn out that "AIDS" is caused by African swine fever virus, Drotman may be sorry that he made such a remark. To say the least, it may leave the CDC open to major multimillion-dollar litigation from swine fever victims and their families.

In the same issue, we reported on a direct mail letter sent out by Jerry Falwell, leader of The Moral Majority, Inc. In it he wrote, "Until recently AIDS was a disease that raged through the male homosexual community, largely because of homosexual promiscuity. But during the last few months, AIDS has begun to infect even larger portions of the general population, heterosexual as well as homosexual. . . . I am going to launch this campaign in Washington and attempt to make strides toward curbing this 'gay plague' as the press calls it." He also wrote, "Over 1 million people are right this minute carrying the AIDS virus, according to medical authorities. You don't have to be gay to get AIDS—anyone can get it."

Falwell went on to bemoan the "innocent" people who had gotten AIDS: "hemophiliacs, unborn children, a transfused nun." He continued, "My friend, if we don't stop this epidemic soon, our entire population could be at risk." After outlining draconian legislative measures that Falwell wanted enacted to stop the epidemic, and asking his readers to send in $15, $25 or $50, he added a P.S.: "I am not persecuting the homosexuals. I pray for their conversion."

Given Jean Dodds's attitude toward me and her rather petulant skepticism about Jane Teas's African swine fever hypothesis, I was dubious about her ability to conduct the necessary research thoroughly and objectively. Where the science of AIDS was concerned, it increasingly struck me that objectivity was in the eye of the beholder.

I must say that the design of the New York State ASFV experiment was quite clever. Instead of testing a large number of AIDS patients for African swine fever virus in a *straightforward* manner, Dodds designed a research project to determine whether HTLV-III and African swine fever were co-factors in AIDS. Instead of testing the Teas hypothesis, they seemed to be disingenuously testing some kind of Dodds's hypothesis. In the *Native* I wrote, "the design of the research project indicates that the hypothesis that AIDS is caused by African swine fever virus may either have been deliberately avoided or at least obfuscated by a faulty research design."

Predictably, the state found no correlation between HTLV-III and African swine fever virus. Out of a total of 160 blood samples tested, only ten were from AIDS patients. That was a ridiculously small number of people to test for a virus which can be difficult to find *even when you know the pigs are infected with it*. Sometimes many different kinds of tests are required to detect ASFV infection. But the state did inadvertently uncover something that was very disturbing.

Out of 110 blood samples from the New York blood supply that were tested, four percent tested positive for African swine fever virus, a virus that the United States Department of Agriculture assured us could not be found anywhere in the continental United States. Actually, the number may have been higher than that because an additional 25 percent of the blood showed some degree of positivity, and if they had been included in the count of positives, the conclusion could have been drawn that 27 percent of the blood in New York's blood banks was infected with African swine fever virus, which could have suggested that there might be a catastrophic epidemic *of some kind* simmering in the general population.

I complained, in a September 30 editorial, that the person who performed the actual testing was not a specialist in the field of African swine fever, and I pointed out that the testing the state did was not thorough. I wrote, "Given that the State Commissioner of Health, David Axelrod, functions under the thumb of the Centers for Disease Control, there may be little that Axelrod will do to pursue the findings. In the past, the head of the AIDS Task Force at the CDC, James

Curran, has expressed a great deal of concern that the pork industry could be affected by the hypothesis that AIDS is caused by African swine fever virus. There is a great deal that the public can do to make sure that their government is protecting them. By demanding that blood banks screen for African swine fever virus, scientists may be forced to face the now very real possibility that the virus is present in the nation's blood supply."

I also expressed my concern that the state did not consult with William Hess as I had recommended to Dodds. Hess had spent much of his life studying African swine fever virus and was working at Plum Island at the time the state was doing its ASFV tests. In a paper on African swine fever in 1981, Hess wrote, "The first diagnosis of ASFV in a country should be based on virus isolated." The state chose to look for antibodies first. Hess also warned in his paper, "No single test can be expected to detect the disease under all conditions." He insisted that only a "comprehensive" battery of tests could be counted on to determine if a pig is infected with ASFV.

I wrote in the *Native,* "If between four and 27 percent of the blood in New York City does indeed contain infectious African swine fever virus, and the public health authorities continue to adhere to the dictates of the pork lobbies and the USDA, the City may be sitting on a time bomb that will make the epidemic to date look quite minor. The governor, the mayor, the city's health commissioner, and the state's health commissioner all have new facts about swine fever's presence in our city's blood supply. Whether they will act in time remains to be seen."

Around the same time that New York State did its testing, Jane Teas and two collaborators, John Beldekas and her husband, James Hebert, had obtained irradiated ASFV from Plum Island so that they themselves could test AIDS blood for the presence of the virus. They had waited months for the USDA to finally comply with their request.

In the course of his ASFV experiments, which were conducted at Boston University, Beldekas also tested the blood from a pig from a local farm. Surprisingly, the pig's blood tested positive for African swine fever virus. When Beldekas notified me, I called the USDA, assuming that alarms would go off, because any discovery of swine fever in pigs in this country would be tantamount to a national agricultural emergency. The day after the USDA was notified, they flew three swine fever experts to Boston to consult with Beldekas. Teas, in a letter to Senator Edward Kennedy about the USDA's visit to

Beldekas, wrote, "During their first visit they indicated to Dr. Beldekas that they have data from slaughterhouses surveys [indicating that] pigs in New York, New Jersey and Texas have been exposed to African swine fever virus. The work of Dr. Beldekas, however, is the first to show the presence of actual virus in a pig from the United States."

Teas wrote to Kennedy because she was afraid that the USDA might prevent Beldekas from continuing the research. She told Kennedy, "Until I began working with Dr. Beldekas, I only wanted to test the idea of whether African swine fever virus causes AIDS. Based on information obtained through a Freedom of Information Act request, and two Congressional inquiries, one conducted by Senator Durenberger and one by Congressman Weiss, I learned that the CDC had done testing on AIDS patients, but had decided that the positives to African swine fever virus must have been mistakes. I do not doubt their right to their opinion, but I strongly object to their decision not to publish their information, along with their methodology and results. I want more from my government than science behind closed doors."

She told Kennedy about her trips to Spain, England, and Uganda in which she attempted to get her hypothesis tested. She wrote about the positive results from England as well as the puzzling problems she encountered in Spain: "I carried duplicate samples of the same AIDS blood to Madrid for testing. Although I had the verbal agreement of the director that the test would be done, when I have called to ask about the results of the tests, the telephone lines have suddenly gone dead when I mention African swine fever virus. Likewise, my letters have gone unanswered."

I figured I had reached the end of the road with the State of New York and after I saw the state commissioner of health saying some bizarre things on television about AIDS, I wrote an angry editorial voicing my frustration in the October 14, 1985, issue of *New York Native*:

> "We continue to find it interesting that the state's Health Commissioner David Axelrod has, as one of his employees, one of the few researchers in the world with swine fever expertise, Jean Dodds, a woman who bragged to us that she was handling the next round of AIDS grants. We also find it interesting that Axelrod is not stopping the transfusion of ASFV-infected blood into unsuspecting New Yorkers.

We had been led to believe that Axelrod is a decent man and a decent scientist. We thought he would be part of the solution of the AIDS epidemic. It turns out he is part of the problem. On a recent telecast of *Inside Albany* (a New York political news show) on October 1, Axelrod talked about AIDS: "This is a behavioral problem," he said. "And I think we have an obligation to help these people and those who become ill as a result of these behavioral activities."

Axelrod clearly had become a hopeless cause and not so different from the gay-behavior-obsessed political epidemiologists who had crafted the AIDS paradigm down at the CDC. Mel Rosen had told me that he and Axelrod used to pray together. Rosen, who was gay (he was a former director of Gay Men's Health Crisis in New York), also told me that Axelrod used to ask him who was gay in Mayor Ed Koch's administration and was very eager to know if Koch himself was gay. Rosen said he liked to tease Axelrod by telling him that he knew who was gay in the administration, and then would refuse to tell him. In many ways Axelrod seemed to be just another public health official pruriently preoccupied with sniffing out gays during the epidemic.

Rosen and I soon stopped speaking and one of the last things he told me was that they had a nickname for me in Albany. They called me "Oink." Rosen himself would eventually die of AIDS. Maybe that wouldn't have happened if the state had done the right thing.

In the October 21 issue, I wrote an editorial about the confusion between CMV, a virus often seen in AIDS, and African swine fever virus: "Here's an open challenge to doctors who read this newspaper. Did you know that CMV (cytomegalovirus) and African swine fever virus, when viewed in thin sections, are morphologically very similar? Did you know that experienced diagnostic laboratories have confused the two in the past? Would you bet your patient's life that you're not confusing the two? Would you bet your own?" When the Centers for Disease Control had first investigated AIDS, they thought the cause might be CMV because it was present in all AIDS patients. They ruled it out because no single strain could be found in all patients. I suspected that they were staring at African swine fever virus and just assuming it was CMV.

In the same issue, I also wrote a story about something very curious

I had learned regarding a possible connection between AIDS and insulin derived from pigs: "A source in the medical community who wishes to remain anonymous has informed the *Native* that there is currently a secret investigation underway to determine whether there is a connection between AIDS and pig insulin." My source had told me that research was being conducted at the Joslin Clinic in Boston, a major diabetes research center, because several people who had received insulin from pigs had gone on to develop AIDS. The director of the clinic denied the story.

Throughout that autumn, I had been trying to get the reporters who helped write Jack Anderson's syndicated column to address the question of whether the government was covering up the connection between AIDS and African swine fever virus. In Anderson's October 7, 1985, column, he reported, "Some medical researchers suspect that the federal government is discouraging tests that might identify a deadly swine virus as a cause of AIDS for fear that such a revelation would wreck the pork industry." Anderson also reported, "Memos reveal that the tests did show a couple of positive reactions, but agricultural researchers dismissed the results as 'false positives.' "

That October, the true political colors of the epidemic started to reveal themselves when Ann Fettner obtained a document on AIDS policy from an influential right-wing think tank called The Free Congress Research and Education Foundation. She described the contents of their document in that same October 21 *Native*:

> AIDS is defined as presenting two types of problems, "behavioral," and "biological." Gay men and drug abusers fall into the first category, and all others with AIDS, "especially the 'unknown' and the blood recipients" into the second, which "poses a health problem of a totally different order; eliminating the biological cause of the problem where the patient's disease was not the result of his own behavior."
>
> A section of the document titled "Gay Rights Dilemma/Agenda Regarding AIDS," includes the following: "At present, homosexuals are faced with two options, either of which is generally unacceptable and therefore unworkable within that political community: 1) give up their sexual practices, a large part of their identity); 2) threaten their newly won civil

rights by continuing their society-threatening behavior. Two courses of action may deliver them from their dilemma: 1) A quick spread of AIDS to the population at large; 2) a quick development of AIDS vaccines. Both will lead to a 'status quo ante' situation. The only way to avoid the homosexual bashing by the 'gay groups' is to frame the whole issue as a public health problem and by identifying homosexuals as 'high-risk' risk-takers with the public health. This approach will help to stop the spread of AIDS, and by that fact, heighten the dilemma."

The document further recommends "education" and "sanctions" for those with "the human behavior problem." These sanctions have to have high visibility and the concurrence of the population, or they will backfire on the education effort and the social pressure effects. Sanctions could have the opposite effect (social protection of the risk-takers) if they are not seen as just and effective. "Given the civic ramifications of AIDS-risking behaviors, a trade-off between civil rights and civic responsibility seems in order here. If this trade-off is publicly acceptable, the sanctions should be the mandatory reporting of all intercourse contacts of the AIDS-riskers."

Among the "sanctions," the document recommends, "for AIDS carriers who are sexually compulsive, make Deprovera optional. Deprovera reduces sex drive." Deprovera, a female hormone which is no longer used in this country due to the suspicion that it causes birth defects, is used in Third-World countries for birth control. Its long-term effects on males are completely unknown.

When Fettner first showed me this document, I felt like I was staring into the abyss. It was like seeing papers from the Wansee conference in Nazi Germany. If there is ever an honest AIDS museum, this document deserves a prominent display. As far as I'm concerned, the document didn't just express the politics of the Reagan White House and its conservative friends. It also was built on the epidemiology of the Reagan CDC which, as would become clearer and clearer, was ignoring the nature of the real epidemic.

Even medical professionals began to sound like the right wing crazies. Scientist John Beldekas wrote an article, for the same issue of the *Native*, about an October 3, 1985 speech by Dr. James O. Mason, the Mormon Director of the Centers for Disease Control: "Dr. Mason of the CDC began his talk with an overview of the epidemic, stressing the idea that behavior is the cause of AIDS. He emphasized male-to-male and female-to-male transmission in both America and Africa, and stated that anal intercourse is the chief mode of transmission. According to Mason the permissive nature of the 1960s and 1970s made the environment ripe for AIDS, and the increase in promiscuity among homosexuals and heterosexuals and increased jet travel introduced the virus into the United States. Mason's idea of behavior as causal . . . was all-pervasive and indicated not only his bias, but attitudes at the highest level of the government. He stressed that casual contact is not a means of transmission, and that the risk of acquiring AIDS in this manner is nonexistent. Mason claimed that 'All people are not at risk for AIDS,' and stated that drastic changes in behavior will be the only way out of the problem. 'High-tech science will not save us from AIDS,' said Mason, 'but changes in behavior will.' "

Beldekas also wrote, "Mason stated that over ten million Africans are infected with the so-called 'AIDS virus,' that AIDS is not a new disease, and that it was introduced into Africa's human population through the eating of green monkey meat or through monkey bites. He claimed that the disease is biologically caused in Africa. This raised the possibility that, if ten million Africans are infected with HTLV-III and if the rate of AIDS is lower there, perhaps HTLV-III is not the cause of AIDS."

Around that time, the serious contradiction in the HTLV-III theory also surfaced in the recommendations about the Elisa test for AIDS which were provided by the American Medical Association. Because the test for HTLV-III was so inaccurate at that point, the AMA had one list of recommendations for "high-risk individuals" with repeated positive results, and a different list of recommendations for "low-risk individuals" with repeated positive test results. A "high-risk" person who tested positive for the virus was to assume that the test result was a true positive, but a "low-risk" [i.e. heterosexual] individual should "be advised about interpretation of these test results. This should include an understanding that the prevalence of false positive results in the low-risk group may be high, and that the patient's particular result may be of questionable significance."

In an October 14 editorial, I wrote, "What all this means is simple. Many positive tests are actually negative and many negative tests are actually positive, and there is no definitive way to discern which tests are true anything. This is a blood test on the basis of which many researchers would like us to make decisions regarding sex, pregnancy, school attendance, marriage, employment, insurance, and other little routine matters of life. The AMA can't tell up from down with this test, yet we are asking Americans to alter the basic social fabric of our culture on the results of the Elisa test."

One of the most articulate and outspoken challengers of the idea that HTLV-III was the cause of AIDS at that time was the previously mentioned Dr. Joseph Sonnabend, who had an eight-year-old practice in Greenwich Village that served gay men. Sonnabend had spent a great many years doing medical research and had assisted the man who discovered interferon. He had extensive experience in cancer research, venereal diseases, and herpes. Sonnabend was critical both of the definition of what AIDS was and of the theory that the single virus, HTLV-III, was the cause of AIDS.

In an interview, in the October 7 issue, Sonnabend had told our reporter Barry Adkins that the CDC "had a very simple-minded way of looking at things." He argued, "The environment in which people with AIDS have been living, or to which they have been exposed, is a complicated microbiological environment in the case of gay men, and that the nature of the exposure is such that you expect multiple diseases, multiple conditions to occur. We know that people with AIDS generally report a much higher frequency of syphilis than people who don't have AIDS. You don't assume that syphilis is a pathway toward AIDS. But to tell you the truth, according to the view that I would have about the development of AIDS, I would say syphilis may indeed contribute to the development of AIDS."

Sonnabend, who was a "multifactorialist," was convinced that AIDS had many causes which interacted "in such a way cumulatively, over a period of time" to produce the syndrome. He complained, "The people researching this disease, the physicians who write in the journals, just see men who have been referred to them. They know nothing about the setting, the overall environment of the patient. They don't look at the disease in the totality."

Sonnabend insisted, "The cause of AIDS is not known—that's the one true thing to say. I have to keep coming back to this. To say that the cause of AIDS is known is cruel. If you say that the cause is known, it means you can go after treatment for the cause and you neglect, unfortunately, not only the other treatments . . . but also research."

Without realizing it at the time, Sonnabend was onto something that linked AIDS to what would ultimately turn out to be the other face of AIDS in the general population—chronic fatigue syndrome. He was convinced that the reactivation of Epstein-Barr virus in AIDS was a major factor in its pathogenesis. In its early days the reactivation of that virus was thought to be the iconic characteristic of chronic fatigue syndrome which initially was called "chronic mono." He told Adkins, "EBV is the virus that causes mononucleosis. The idea is to consider the known factors in the environment of people who got sick. The ones where we know and understand the effects, and to ask how these could interact and combine to produce AIDS. One factor is the reactivation of a good number of such agents—EBV, CMV, HTLV-III. HTLV-III may be no more than another virus reactivated by the true cause of AIDS. There is no evidence that would say differently."

Sonnabend was not afraid to name names (which got him occasionally into political trouble): "Unlike what Dr. Anthony Fauci [the head of the National Institute of Allergy and Infectious Diseases (NIAID)] and Dr. Robert Gallo tell us, we are very far from understanding this disease. Very little is known. The sort of smugness that emanates from the government scientists is offensive, considering what's at stake and what is happening now. The only people who are pleased over this are the ones who've received millions of dollars' worth of support, and these are the government scientists and big medical centers and also people who really, I think, have missed the boat, who have an inordinate influence on media accessibility and are responsible, along with many others, for the panic that's going on now—and the disaster."

Sonnabend was from the school that believed the single virus theory was actually a ploy to take away the onus from the gay lifestyle—a theory that I have argued is also "homodemiological" and an essentially ironic betrayal of the gay community by a gay doctor. He told Adkins, "It's easier to say, bad luck, a virus hit. That's another reason why people might have favored the single virus theory. In the fullness of time, however, the virus did come, and we find the gay men who wanted it so much, now they've got it. And what they've also got is quarantine, and in fact the very thing they were fighting for is not so wonderful." Why Sonnabend thought his own gay lifestyle theory was so helpful to the gay community always somehow escaped me throughout the epidemic. His absurd kind of loose talk (based on even looser reasoning) about what gay men *wanted* to be the cause, was very strange. That gay men, who, at that time, were basically chickens running around with their political heads cut off, could be accused of such a conscious monocausal conspiracy was a real stretch.

What was interesting about the way Sonnabend argued about causation was that it always questioned the motives of the theorizers and the social implications of the theory. One was held responsible for the political consequences of one's ideas about the cause of AIDS. At the time Sonnabend was open-minded about the possible involvement of African swine fever virus in AIDS, but not very enthusiastic because it too was *a single-virus theory* and hence it was—in his mind—politically dangerous. Sonnabend's thinking was typical of an environment in which one could easily be intimidated from telling the truth because the consequences of the inconvenient truth might be too horrible. I was getting very frustrated by this kind of thinking that had a strong whiff of emotional blackmail. I thought the only way out of the epidemic was through discovering and telling the raw factual truth without regard to political consequences. I didn't think politics would save a single patient if there was not a commitment to unvarnished, scientific facts and medical truth. I couldn't even bring up African swine fever virus to Sonnabend without him suggesting it was an idea that would lead to quarantine.

Because Sonnabend did not buy the government's party line on HTLV-III, he was gradually elbowed out of an AIDS organization and an AIDS journal that he had help start. The AIDS Medical Foundation, which he started with millionairess and scientific researcher Mathilde Krim, moved toward an alliance with the HTLV-III establishment at Harvard and the National Cancer Institute. Sonnabend resigned when the organization sent out an alarming press release by Terry Beirn, a man with a public relations background that Sonnabend had hired as the administrative director. The press release said, "Nobody is now safe from AIDS, it's on the loose." Sonnabend was offended that the press release suggested that AIDS was being casually transmitted. It broke Sonnabend's don't-scare-the-horses rule.

After his break from the Krim organization, Sonnabend grew increasingly dissatisfied with what Mathilde Krim was saying publicly about the epidemic and privately mocked her rather uptight and puritanical attitude toward sex. What I didn't like about her organization was that it was a private organization that took money from well-meaning people and then used it to basically back research into the exact same ideas that the government was promoting about AIDS. Over the years it increasingly seemed to me to be a very big part of the problem of the real epidemic rather than a solution. Her organization had essentially privatized the Big Assumption.

In the October 28 issue of *New York Native,* Ann Fettner wrote a piece about Douglas Feldman, a medical anthropologist who taught at New York University. He had visited the small African country of Rwanda in order to investigate its AIDS epidemic. Fettner reported that Feldman told her, "While green monkey skins are used for clothing, the animals aren't eaten (as alleged by the Centers for Disease Control head James O. Mason). About 20 percent of the population, however, eats pork when it's available. In the south around Butari, there is no pork left. All the pigs died about two years ago." He also said, "There was an epizootic in the south central region near Butari which has not been identified as to its cause," and "While I'm sure HTLV-III/LAV is necessary to AIDS, I'm not at all convinced that it is alone sufficient to cause this syndrome. I definitely have questions about differences in the rate of AIDS and antibody positives between the two areas of Rwanda. The death of pigs really has to be looked at now."

Even as it became clearer and clearer that HTLV-III was not the cause of AIDS, the social and biomedical agenda was proceeding throughout 1985 as though it was an incontrovertible fact. A new kind of professional was emerging: "the HTLV-III counselor." Orwell would have loved it. These were paid busybodies who would "educate" (that is "re-educate") people on how to live their lives if they tested positive for a virus that had not been shown to cause AIDS—by a highly unreliable test. Congress was only too willing to pay for this propaganda campaign. Senator Patrick Moynihan announced he wanted to spend 25 million dollars on "public education" about AIDS. "Public education" is one excellent way to keep the conventional wisdom of science carved in stone. "Public education" is one way to discredit and stigmatize doubt and dissidence.

Unfortunately, most so-called gay leaders were on the same page as the government. In the July 29 issue, I wrote an editorial about the director of the National Gay Task Force, titled, "Jeff Levi, the Nightmare":

> Anyone who reads this newspaper knows that there are many researchers who can't get sufficient money to do important research into treatments for AIDS. A conspiracy-minded person might actually see a deliberate attempt to create a medieval situation that will evoke draconian medieval solutions.
>
> We know that "treatment" is a dirty word for God's spokespeople on the New Right, and apparently a matter of indifference to the director of the Centers for Disease Control. We also know that the level of funding for research at the federal and state level, given the enormity of this public health problem, constitutes a sick joke.
>
> So what does Senator Daniel Patrick Moynihan propose to do? Instead of proposing a commitment of 25 million dollars for treatment research, he proposes the commitment of 25 million dollars for public education. How can anyone be against public education? It's as American as Mom and apple pie. And that's exactly our point: public education for a syndrome like AIDS often comes down to throwing mom and apple pie at a problem which should be addressed through vigorous research and by declaring a scientific war on the virus itself. Destabilize the virus, not American sexuality. Public education on AIDS comes down to a war against sex, and guess who always wins that one?
>
> According to Mark Bernstein of Moynihan's office, two of the biggest proponents of the legislation are Dr. James Curran of the CDC, who has botched everything he's touched for four years, and Jeff Levi, the acting director of The National Gay Task Force. Levi thinks that changing the sexual behavior of gay men is what NGTF should be doing to deal with the epidemic. Gay men got the message on that years ago. Levi should be demanding the development of serious, effective treatment for AIDS instead of falling into the New

Right trap of using prevention as a way of keeping America zipped up for Biblical reasons.

Bogus public education may win Jeff Levi a mom and apple pie constituency in D.C., but the rest of us, hopefully, can see though his antics. Levi may become a major New Right hero as the man who destroyed NGTF.

A clear picture of what was really happening was starting to form in my mind. In the August 11 issue, I went even further, in another editorial, titled "The United States of AIDS":

> As things stand, the basic public health plan is to create a two-tier system in America of the sero-negative and the seropositive. All will be *counseled*. The seronegatives will be counseled to stay away from the time bombs.
>
> Thus, there will be no freedom from AIDS. Either you will have it, or you will be in danger of getting it. A disease has been found with which to forge the most diabolical program of sexual control yet conceived by the very clever fascistic types in the public health service in collusion with God knows who else.
>
> Life will cease to be life as we know it. It will be lived under the aegis of "protection and control" guidelines. One will not think of oneself as a human being, but as a member of a "risk group," a kind of caste with the biological mark of Cain. If one is gay, one will always be guilty of not "changing one's behavior" or "reducing one's risk" until proven innocent. And no matter how high the percentage of gay people who do buy into the "prevention and control" is, there will always be some auto-homophobic voice on a *Phil Donahue* show to say, "Oh, no, my friends haven't changed at all—they're still promiscuous." And "Tsk, tsk, you just can't change homosexuals through education." Then will come the attempts at treating the behavior itself, Soviet-style.
>
> It's time for gay Americans to think of "counseling programs" as a kind of parole, and AIDS counselors as

"parole officers." These people are the vehicles of sexual control. . . . They are the benign face of an evil social strategy that has been devised to put the gay community back in its place.

Only our deepest evolutionary political instincts will get us out of this one. Any heroes out there? Start creating new gay institutions. Don't get suckered into the National Gay Task Force or the Gay Men's Health Crisis approach to things. There are good and bad things about both organizations. But we need many more individually tailored, imaginative approaches to fight the New Right agenda on AIDS. And where are the Goddamned gay intellectuals?

I was to learn over the next quarter of a century that the phrase "gay intellectual" was kind of an oxymoron, at least where the epidemic was concerned. Those who could deconstruct Sondheim were not necessarily also able to decipher the horrific reality of the situation around them that had covertly transformed their community into biomedical dystopia. As Hannah Arendt said about Nazi Germany, "The purely personal problem was not what your enemies were doing but what your friends were doing."

Also in the August 11, 1985 issue, John Lauritsen, a Harvard-educated research analyst, who eventually wrote around 50 articles for *New York Native*, explored the role of poppers in AIDS. He reported, "Poppers are a liquid mixture of isobutyl nitrite and other chemicals, packaged in small bottles under such names as 'Rush,' 'Ram,' 'Thunderbolt,' 'Locker Room,' and 'Crypt Tonight.' . . . When inhaled just before orgasm, poppers seem to enhance and prolong the sensation. With regular use, poppers become a sexual crutch, and many gay men are incapable of having sex, even masturbation, without the aid of poppers. . . . In 1981, the Stanford Medical Laboratories tested different brands of poppers and found them to contain kerosene, hydrochloric acid, and sulfur dioxide, among other impurities."

Lauritsen criticized the FDA for not regulating poppers as a drug. They were allowed to be sold as room odorizers. In 1985, they were declared illegal. Lauritsen argued in the *Native* that scientists had known about the toxic effects of poppers for many years. Lauritsen did his own epidemiological survey: "In Massachusetts, where poppers have been banned for years, only 178 cases of AIDS had been reported as of May 6, 1985. In contrast there had been 3,756 cases in New York State, where poppers were sold legally in sex shops, baths, discos, and even smoke shops until this June." For Lauritsen, there was no question that poppers were involved in AIDS; the question was how much of a factor were they? He argued, "96-100 percent of the gay men with AIDS used poppers, usually quite heavily. These men were also heavy users of other 'recreational' drugs including amphetamines, cocaine, heroin, Quaaludes, LSD, barbituates, and ethyl chloride." He pointed to a study that had concluded that all men who had Kaposi's sarcoma had been poppers users and another study that correlated poppers use with immunological abnormalities. In one study of mice exposed to poppers, all the mice died. Another study showed that the T-4 cells which are depleted in AIDS patients could also be depleted by exposure to poppers. One of the things that poppers are capable of causing was cardiovascular collapse. Lauritsen mocked a local group of gay doctors called Physicians for Human Rights, who urged gay men not to use poppers or other recreational drugs because they could "impair your judgment." Even discussions about drug use had to be framed around the so-called AIDS virus, rather than the damage the drugs could do to the body all by themselves.

1986: A New Virus or a Renamed Old One?

By early 1986, the CDC was beginning to urge people—especially gay people—to be tested for antibodies to HTLV-III. James Curran, the director of the AIDS Task Force, visited New York on January 6 and called for massive HTLV-III testing because it was "the most important infection in the U.S. in adults." In our article on the matter, Barry Adkins reported, "Gay Men's Health Crisis Executive Director Richard Dunne and AIDS researcher Dr. John Beldekas of Boston University both told the *Native* there is no evidence to support Curran's conclusion." In the same *Native* article, Adkins also reported, "Curran said anyone who truly tests positive to LAV/HTLV-III antibody is infected with the virus. He explained that the virus is very difficult to isolate, and one third of those antibody-positive cases in which virus is not isolated are basically a fluke. Curran maintains that these people are actually infected. Dunne and Beldekas later told the *Native* that Curran's statements were inherently homophobic. Disagreeing with Curran's statistics, Dunne said that in 40 percent of antibody-positive cases, the virus is unable to be isolated. Beldekas explained that in order to isolate the virus from lymphocytes, scientists must create an 'artificial in vitro condition,' which is then manipulated by various drugs, creating an unnatural situation. According to Beldekas, there is no clinical data to support Curran's theory, and Curran is making a 'quantum leap from antibody to infection.' " Curran also told Adkins that while he had some problems with contact tracing, he would not necessarily rule it out as an option. At that point the New York City Health Department said there were no plans for HTLV-III contact tracing.

During that same period, the Texas Board of Health was considering measures to quarantine people with AIDS, "if he or she has certain circumstances which create a threat to the public health if not immediately controlled." In an interview with the *Native*'s John Fall, published in the January 20, 1986, issue, the Texas commissioner of Health, Dr. Robert Bernstein, said that a quarantine person with AIDS who was still "having sex with the public would remain in medical isolation until this behavior changes."

Among the media organizations in 1986, the *New York Native* was virtually alone in questioning the orthodox notion that HTLV-III was the cause of AIDS. The lockstep that would characterize the media during the epidemic had begun. Even the *Village Voice*, which most people erroneously think of as anti-establishment and pro-gay, adopted an aggressive policy of trusting and supporting the government's scientific pronouncements about the epidemic. (Most people forget that the *Village Voice* actually had to be dragged kicking and screaming into its support of gay civil rights issues.) Early that year a *Village Voice* writer named Anna Mayo tried to start writing critically about AIDS, but she was discouraged by a gay writer at the *Village Voice* named Richard Goldstein. She called me at the *Native* and told me that she had written an article on AIDS called "The Principle of Uncertainty," which her editor at the *Voice*, Robert Friedman, was refusing to publish. She also told me that Goldstein was trying to manipulate the situation at the paper so that she would never write about AIDS. While I hadn't agreed with many of Mayo's ideas on AIDS, the suppression of her writing concerned me. I agreed to publish the article, and on the March 10 *Native* cover, we showed a bound-and-gagged woman in a *Village Voice* T-shirt with the headline, "The Article the *Village Voice* Suppressed Begins on Page 15."

Mayo's piece was a look at several alternative theories about the cause of AIDS. She examined Dr. Ernest Sternglass's hypothesis that AIDS is caused by "interactive exposure to radiation during the nuclear weapons tests in the 1950s and '60s." She reported on Sternglass's visit to an AIDS conference in Europe at which he presented his ideas to Robert Gallo. Sternglass told Mayo that Gallo had eventually taken him seriously, but Mayo had her doubts: "Gallo come around? I didn't believe it for a minute. Gallo works for the National Cancer Institute, one of the National Institutes of Health (NIH). Any halfway smart government scientist knows enough not to propose an investigation of radiation effects. (If you work for the nuclear state, you sign an unwritten nuclear loyalty oath.) And Gallo could have other motives for not subscribing to Sternglass's theory. It could appear to him as a challenge to the dogma that AIDS is caused by HTLV-III, which Gallo claims to have discovered. . . . Gallo sits on the review committees for grants and makes recommendations for government jobs and contracts to private industry. He's said to hanker after a Nobel Prize for discovering the cause of AIDS. But what if some other virus were shown to be the cause of AIDS and HTLV-III were reduced to the status of a mere marker? Prizes might slip from Gallo's grasp."

Mayo interviewed Gallo, who told her that at first he thought Sternglass was just another "nut." But he said that later in the evening he realized that Sternglass was a serious person, but didn't know anything about AIDS. Predictably, Gallo yelled at Mayo, "HTLV-III is the sole cause of AIDS! There's no question about it. You don't need any cofactors. It gives you AIDS all alone." Then came my favorite part of her article: "His [Gallo's] tone turned ugly. 'This guy Sternglass sounds like Chuck Ortleb, the editor of the *New York Native*. Do you realize Ortleb has actually persuaded the government to spend money on this ridiculous swine flu [sic] idea?' Gallo continued, 'At first I thought Ortleb must be mentally off, but I talked to some gay leaders in New York—no, I can't say who—and they explained to me that he is just out to make money selling newspapers. Now I can understand that mentality, but I don't want to have anything to do with that sort of journalist. You're not one of them, are you?' "

In the same article, Mayo examined the fact that HTLV-III had not fulfilled Koch's postulates, which are generally accepted as necessary to prove that an organism causes a disease. She pointed out that a high percentage of AIDS patients do not have HTLV-III in their blood, and that health care workers who had become infected with the virus had not developed the disease. She also explored the African swine fever virus hypothesis. She quoted Jane Teas as saying, "I think HTLV-III may be an endogenous virus. That is, in a latent state, it has been present in most of us from birth. When swine fever or some other virus weakens the immune system, HTLV-III appears."

Mayo also examined the theory that the use of oral recreational drugs was the original cause of AIDS, as well as the Sonnabend theory that repeated viral infections weakened the immune system. She also brought up the Belle Glade, Florida researcher, Dr. Mark Whiteside's idea that HTLV-III was just a marker for AIDS. He thought the disease was caused by an insect-borne arbovirus. He told Mayo, "In Belle Glade where they have neither homosexuality nor heterosexual promiscuity, the disease is passed by insects that breed in open sewers and at night enter windows that have neither screen nor glass."

When we asked for a comment from the *Village Voice* editor, about the failure to publish Mayo's piece, Robert Friedman told us, "I felt that the end product was too speculative. It didn't convince me. The alternative theories [presented] did not completely undercut the HTLV-III [case], which I'm not particularly wedded to myself. It is well-written and entertaining. I just had qualms about printing it."

One of the jobs of future historians of the epidemic will be to try and track down all the articles critical of the AIDS establishment that were not published because of editorial "qualms."

Three years after she first proposed the hypothesis that AIDS is caused by African swine fever virus, Jane Teas succeeded in testing her hypothesis in an American laboratory. With her husband, epidemiologist James Hebert, and Boston University researcher John Beldekas, she obtained viral testing materials from the U.S. Department of Agriculture. It was only because the press (mostly the *Native*) had taken an interest in the matter that the USDA cooperated. Teas, Beldekas, and Hebert used two kinds of tests to detect African swine fever in AIDS sera: one called hemadsorption technique and one called direct immunofluorescence. They tested the blood of 21 people with AIDS, 12 with lymphadenopathy and 16 controls. Using the direct immunofluorescence test, ten of the 21 AIDS patients, 4 of the people with lymphadenopathy, and one of the 16 controls tested positive. The team submitted their results, in the form of a letter, to the British Medical Journal, *The Lancet*, and the letter was published on March 8, 1986. The authors concluded that they had "found evidence consistent with African swine fever virus (ASFV) infection in the plasma of U.S. patients with Acquired Immunodeficiency Syndrome (AIDS) and lymphadenopathy syndrome." They were cautious about the interpretation of their findings: "The results of these various tests suggest the presence of a hitherto unknown virus in these cell cultures. ASFV has not been thought to be infectious to humans or known to occur in U.S. swine. Therefore, these results point either to an anomaly of the testing procedures by cross-reactivity with some unknown AIDS-associated virus, or they suggest a new variant of ASFV that is infectious to people." The Teas team criticized the prior testing that had been reported on in *The Lancet* because the "sample sizes were very small (seven and eight patients), sera were only examined for antibodies. Since ASFV infects only an estimated 1 percent of macrophages at any one time, large sample sizes, special target assay systems, and several tests may be required to show an effect if a true relationship between ASFV and AIDS exists."

"Is the Reign of Error Over?" was the headline we gave the story about their research on the March 17 cover of the *Native*. In the article I wrote about their findings, I brought up the issue of potential litigation which may have caused some of the hesitation in researching the connection between African swine fever virus and AIDS: "One possible issue of medical liability may involve the recommendation that the USDA makes when a country is exterminating its pigs [because of ASFV]. The recommendations include urging people to consume the infected pigs to speed up the disposal process. A USDA source told us that many Brazilian newspapers told people not to eat pigs infected with African swine fever virus, for fear that human illness would result. The *Native* has also been told by another source in touch with a retired American meat industry executive that there have been three outbreaks of African swine fever in the United States, in the 1940s, the 1950s, and the early 1970s. The retired executive told the *Native* that the outbreaks were described as a different disease at the time. The unnamed USDA official further told the *Native* that one additional problem which is occurring around swine fever is that the Animal Plant Health Inspection Service, the agency responsible for detecting the presence of swine fever, now lacks the competence to detect the disease in the United States."

I also underlined the fact that we had been told that the USDA had data from slaughterhouse surveys of pigs to indicate that pigs in New York, New Jersey, and Texas has been exposed to African swine fever virus. I also wrote that the question before Congress and the media should be "whether the Centers for Disease Control has been aware of the connection between AIDS and African swine fever since the inception of the AIDS epidemic. Because African swine fever resembles cytomegalovirus (CMV) in appearance, it is possible the CDC made an honest error. The CDC has informed the *Native* that their antibody testing for African swine fever virus in 1983 had negative results. But a memo [about the tests] obtained from a CDC file could more accurately be described as inconclusive. Of 16 AIDS patients from San Francisco, three showed some positive reactions for antibody to the virus. A USDA official who asked not to be named has told the *Native* that such results merited additional testing. USDA literature warns that cautious and thorough testing must be done on herds of pigs for African swine fever virus. In pigs, African swine fever virus has sometimes been misdiagnosed as porcine CMV as well as several other diseases. A manual on African swine fever virus contains the following warning: 'Even with good samples, no single test is sufficient. . . . For instance, accurate diagnosis for the acute and chronic phases of African Swine Fever require different tests. In addition, it's now felt that different strains of the virus exist, which are not detected by every test.' "

I again reminded *Native* readers that Judy Petsonk, a reporter for *South Jersey Courier Post*, had interviewed the CDC's James Curran and he had told her "he was afraid that Teas's theory might make people afraid to eat pork, thus harming the pork industry in the United States."

In April, one of our readers sent me a clipping of a column by Ben Stein that appeared in the March 25 issue of the *Los Angeles Herald Examiner*. I suspected that historians would look back on the column as perhaps the first time a journalist inadvertently had picked up on the fact that a chronic form of African swine fever was manifesting itself as an illness in the general population that was eventually called "chronic fatigue syndrome." If it was ASFV, it was spreading throughout the human population in America in exactly the way you would expect it to, manifesting itself in a wide variety of ways as it wrought evolving multisystemic pathologies on its new vulnerable human population. Stein wrote that it seemed to him that everyone in Los Angeles seemed to be sick at the time. People would develop a flu which lasted two weeks and then they would recover. But then a few weeks later they would get sick again. He described "a vague, spaced-out feeling, chronic fatigue just over your shoulder, always breathing down on you, a susceptibility to wild upsets of the bowels all became part of daily life." Stein complained that even though an incurable flu seemed to be spreading throughout Los Angeles, no one was doing anything about it. Public health officials were silent. (That silence would become deafening over the next three decades.)

Stein also wrote, "Already my friends in the East tell me the non-stop flu has hit Washington and New York in a big way. This nation can be genuinely disabled by these incurable diseases. The individuals who have them are severely pained, physically and psychically. Having the flu half your life hurts, take it from me. Can anyone help? Isn't this worthy of national attention? Are we just going to have the stock market go up forever while everyone gets incurable viruses? I'm scared."

In an editorial on Stein's article, in the April 14 issue of *New York Native*, I wrote, "We have warned the Centers for Disease Control, New York State Health Commissioner David Axelrod, the City of New York, gay leaders, Congressmen Ted Weiss and Henry Waxman, and several members of the scientific press about the implications of finding African swine fever in 'AIDS' patients. Any sober expert on swine fever would immediately worry out loud that 'AIDS' is just the tip of the swine fever iceberg and that the virus doesn't select hosts by means of their sexual proclivities, and the disease would be much more widespread in the general population in a matter of time. . . . Swine fever doesn't only cause 'AIDS' in pigs. It can cause chronic respiratory problems for life. And swine fever is not spread only through the kinds of sex that give the geniuses at the Centers for Disease Control hard-ons and hate-ons."

I also reminded our readers about the positive ASFV results that turned up in the New York State testing of blood from blood donors in New York City: "In this population the African swine fever virus antibody is present in 4.5% (5 out of 110) of the population. Moreover, 26 blood samples from that group had what is called 'atypical fluorescence,' which the state did not consider positive. We've said before that they may be playing with fire, because these results suggest to us that African swine fever may be presently infecting the general population of New York City." I concluded my piece by stating, "I certainly wouldn't like to be the one to have to tell the people of Los Angeles that the result of the cover-up of the connection between AIDS and African swine fever is that the entire city of Los Angeles is running around infected with a chronic pig disease. Those people who laugh about our exposé of the swine fever cover-up may soon have to look elsewhere for a chuckle."

"Soon" of course turned out to be another example of my excessive optimism.

It took me a while to track down Ben Stein on the phone. When I finally reached him in Malibu and explained what I thought was going on, he seemed polite enough. But several weeks later he wrote a nasty piece in the right wing publication called *The American Spectator* which, without naming me, mocked me and the things I had told him. He also misrepresented what I had said to him on the phone.

We reported, in the same issue, on a documentary which was filmed by WGBH of Boston as part of its Frontline series. The documentary's filmmakers had followed a man with AIDS who was destitute and dying. The man continued to have sex after he was diagnosed with AIDS. It was a highly inflammatory film which clearly was meant to turn the public against people with AIDS and like most of what was written or said on TV during that period, was meant to equate the AIDS epidemic with the gay citizenry. In a story in the *Native* by Allen Barnett and Barry Adkins, Richard Dunne of Gay Men's Health Crisis said it was "the single worst media representation of gay in recent years." He also said, "You don't frame a discussion of public policy around one aberrant example. People will walk away from this program thinking that this man was spreading AIDS. The program will only lead to discussion of quarantine, for that is the only point of reference in the film."

The film, which was made in gay-friendly Texas, focused on a twenty-year-old man named Fabian Bridge, an African-American man who was warned by gay people in Houston not to have anything to do with the film crew. Sue Lowell, the head of the Gay Political Caucus in Houston, told our reporters, "The film crew left town and left a lapful of problems in a town where gay activists are overworked." She also told *New York Native* that the controversy inspired the Texas Commissioner of Public Health to attempt to gain authority to implement quarantine-like measures in isolated cases. That was the constructive way the media worked with public health authorities during the epidemic. Even the so-called liberal media.

In that same issue of the *Native,* Anne-Christine d'Adesky began a two-part series called "Haiti: The Great AIDS Cover-Up." She reported that, two months after Jean-Claude "Baby Doc" Duvalier was overthrown, doctors began to freely discuss how they had been kept from speaking publicly about the true nature of the AIDS epidemic in that country. She reported that AIDS was actually first diagnosed in Haiti in 1978, *putting it closer to the time that African swine fever broke out in pigs in that country.* For a proper historical reconstruction of the true nature of the AIDS epidemic, it was of great interest that she noted the majority of those with AIDS in Haiti "do not fall into any Centers for Disease Control defined 'high risk' category. Only 40% could have gotten AIDS from bisexual contact (for men) or as blood transfusion (mostly women). Only 10% have Kaposi's sarcoma (KS), while 40% have tuberculosis (mycobacterium TB) or other opportunistic infections. In addition, a higher percentage of women have AIDS in Haiti than in the U.S., and some say that they may pass it on to men."

An organization called GHESKIO, a Haitian study group on Kaposi's sarcoma and opportunistic infections, that had been formed in 1982 in collaboration with doctors at Cornell University in New York, may have inadvertently provided evidence that HTLV-III was not the cause of AIDS. According to d'Adesky, "GHESKIO used the ELISA test to verify presence of HTLV-III antibodies in people's blood. 40% of the patients tested were negative." This should have alerted authorities in our own country that something was seriously wrong with the HTLV-III hypothesis, but unfortunately the etiological train had left the station.

In the following issue of the *Native*, d'Adesky continued her report from Haiti with a story about a former political figure in Haiti who, during the pig eradication program, had been hiding pigs in his home, suggesting that African swine fever may never have been fully eradicated from pigs in that country. It left open the possibility that if ASFV was the actual source of AIDS, that there were still porcine reservoirs of virus that could endanger human health.

On April 21, the *New York Native* published one of its most revealing pieces on the real nature of the fake epidemiology that the CDC was then doing on AIDS and the same kind of epidemiology they would eventually do on chronic fatigue syndrome. "A Place to Die and a Drink of Water," by Ann Fettner, asked, "why the CDC was studying AIDS in Belle Glade when they've already decided to ignore the facts." The CDC investigated the epidemic in the small, poverty-stricken Florida community in order to put to rest the suspicion that AIDS was spread in ways that the CDC had not informed the public about. Fettner described the investigation in a brutal, uncompromising manner: "In lockstep with local health authorities, the CDC is busy predetermining exactly the results it will find in the four-month epidemiological survey currently underway. This is cosmetics, a public relations initiative to rescue the town's reputation while furthering the CDC's control over the shaping of the epidemic. Epidemiology it isn't. They're after sexual and drug use transmission, and any evidence of an unusual cofactor will be sidestepped."

According to Fettner, what the CDC didn't like was "too many non-identifiable risk (NIR) cases" of AIDS which threatened their prevailing paradigm. The CDC wouldn't believe people who said that did not fit into the official gay or drug-taking risk groups. Darlene Lee, the Chief Nursing Officer at a clinic in Belle Glade, made fun of the CDC's sex and drug presumptions to Fettner: " 'There's something about their lifestyles that they're hiding, you keep getting that. They're all closet homosexuals or shooting up,' she says sarcastically. 'We have 25 people right now who're in their 50s and 60s; nowhere else are they seeing these 50- and 60-year-olds, and I'm saying, Sure! They're turning tricks on the side!' "

Fettner reported, "When the CDC surveyed 250 people from the poor southwest neighborhood in Belle Glade, the overall rate was 8% positive. Belle Glade proper was 11% positive in the CDC pilot study, and 60% of all the positives had no risk factors." What a high percentage of the patients did have, according to Fettner, was a significant percentage of insect-borne viruses. Mark Whiteside, a physician who treated patients in Belle Glade told Fettner, "It's incredible that we should still be arguing about NIR [No Identifiable Risk] cases . . . . The disease is not explained by heterosexual transmission in the NIR patients, none of whom have had sex with members of so-called high-risk groups. . . . We're seeing non-characteristic disease and in general it's not explained by heterosexual transmission. For example, I have a 56-year-old woman who has been married for 27 years to her 77-year-old husband. He's healthy, exonerative for HTLV-III. They've had no outside sexual contact—none, zero—and she now has AIDS manifested by disseminated histoplasmosis. Her only chance for a risk is a blood transfusion in 1981." But Fettner reported they tracked all the donors and they were negative for the virus. Interestingly, Whiteside told Fettner "She lives in the same apartment as two other AIDS cases, including one of our original NIR cases, a 30-some-year-old who had fewer than ten lifetime sexual partners and had lived with a woman for seven years—and the woman is still healthy. He's dead."

The health care workers who were seeing inconvenient things the CDC didn't want people to know about were treated in the way most people were when they came in contact with any of the abnormal science of the epidemic. The nurse, Darlene Lee, said, "Everything is fine as long as you don't make waves. You do as you're told and as long as you comply with everything they want, it's okay. But when you're a little bit independent or start asking questions—or God forbid, you do something on your own and try to help these people!" Whiteside and his colleague, according to Fettner, were "perceived by the CDC as an annoyance, objects of ridicule because of their insistence that more is going on in Belle Glade than is explained by the CDC party line. The two physicians had done a door-to-door survey and came up "with 9% positive for HTLV-III, and most did not have an identifiable risk factor."

In her *Native* piece on Belle Glade, Fettner also reported the shocking story of Gus Sermos who had been a CDC surveillance officer for two-and-one-half years in Florida. When Sermos started to raise some serious questions about what was going on in the CDC's

AIDS efforts in Florida, it inspired an investigative series of articles in the *Miami Herald*, and he was punished by being summarily transferred back to a temporary assignment at the CDC's headquarters in Atlanta, in what appeared to be a humiliating demotion. Sermos had suggested that CDC AIDS funds were not being properly used. He told Fettner that while on the job in Florida, he had "uncovered fraud and mismanagement, cavalier attitudes on the part of the CDC, and general lying and cheating." He also told Fettner, "They hired me to do surveillance, but I found out that wasn't what they wanted at all. They didn't want to know anything about what's going on. [CDC AIDS officials] Curran or Jaffe come down and all they want to talk about is fishing, not AIDS. When I started in Florida, I had one supervisor. Then there were two, then three—this raft of people doing nothing but waiting for my reports to come in."

But those Sermos reports were not appreciated. According to Fettner, he said it was like, "I was digging manure and putting it on their plates." He told her, "90% of what they're doing up in Atlanta is public relations. For AIDS there're four people in the field and 40 in Atlanta. If all they're doing with AIDS is lying about it, creating subterfuge, then why not disband them? He described the scientists working on AIDS with Curran and Jaffe in Atlanta as "a bunch of kids right out of medical school, because it's politically so unhealthy to get involved with the CDC AIDS Task Force that older doctors with experience don't want anything to do with it."

One of the epidemiologically embarrassing things that Sermos uncovered in his surveillance was the presence of older people in Florida who had AIDS *without risk factors*, which was clearly a threat to the CDC's AIDS paradigm. Sermos was accused of not asking strong enough questions to prove that the people really did belong in the CDC's politically crafted risk groups. He told Fettner, "I'll tell you the truth, in my wildest dreams I would never have thought they'd get away with what those guys have gotten away with as far as just being, if nothing else, just being bad showmen. And for forgetting that the show has any substance. Basically it's like an old vaudeville show that's been running too long. I can't believe that house of cards in Atlanta can just stand up and take all the wind. But boy, evidently—I've told my wife and I hate admitting it—but they are totally impervious to anything. If you say something disagreeable, you're either unpatriotic or you're a kook. . . . I'm like a citizen who sees a robber running out of the store and calls the cops, and the police arrest you and lock you up for reporting a crime. I wasn't going to be a whore for them; I felt like I was a guard at Auschwitz, a traitor. But they're traitors to their profession and [James] Curran [head of the CDC's Task Force on AIDS] is not a scientist by any definition. He should be selling cars like his father."

What is so uncanny about his story is that his description of the CDC's behavior in the investigation of AIDS would be echoed in everything the CDC eventually did in its fake investigation of chronic fatigue syndrome. The fact that the CDC was able to behave this way for three decades shows that powerful institutional forces were keeping Sermos's so-called house of cards safely in place. It may have seemed like a "vaudeville" act, but we have to remind ourselves that there were those in Germany who didn't think the Nazi leaders would amount to much because they resembled clowns.

What made these Sermos revelations so historically important was that for the first time word was publicly coming from *an insider* that there was something rotten in Denmark. People on the outside with growing doubts about the integrity of the CDC and its story about AIDS were *not crazy*. Everything about what happened to him lends support to the notion that what could be called totalitarian or abnormal science (as well as "homodemiology") had already become the official culture of AIDS. The CDC didn't want to know what was really going on. Or they did know all too well and they didn't want the public to know the truth. To borrow a notion from Hannah Arendt, they had manufactured a false epidemiological image of what was going on and used powerful public relations resources to make it the conventional wisdom for America and the rest of the world. An honest, courageous man warned the world from inside the belly of a authoritarian beast that public health had turned itself into something evil. His reference to "Auschwitz" was downright prophetic.

In the April 28 issue of *New York Native,* Fettner again addressed the quality of the CDC's epidemiology. She wrote, "The days I spent recently in Belle Glade, Florida, have left an even more sour taste in my mouth than usual over the mishandling and manipulation of the AIDS epidemic by the federal Centers for Disease Control in Atlanta. Because there can be little question that the two tenured AIDS experts down there, Drs. James Curran and Harold Jaffe, have insufficient stature to be guiding such important matters, it's obviously been someone like Dr. James Mason (who you may recall served as acting

Assistant Secretary for Health and Human Services while still head of the CDC, and who is back in Atlanta now) who's running the show, with directions from someone near the President or whoever does his AIDS-thinking for him)." Any definitive understanding of the history of the epidemic will ultimately have to take a close forensic look at the chain of command in the White House and the source(s) of that political "AIDS-thinking." She also wrote, "The function of the CDC is to do epidemiology. One wonders if they know what that means. Originally 'epidemiology' meant the study of epidemics, but its definition has grown broader and includes tracking outbreaks of poisonings, keeping track of non-communicable diseases, and developing statistics about the whos, wheres, and hows of such as automobile fatalities, mental illness, cancer, and communicable diseases. Basically, one can sum up the function of epidemiology in three major variables: Person, Place and Time. When it comes to communicable diseases, there are certainties about each that need to be known. The CDC long ago exhausted its imagination by designating the Person category to gays, junkies, hookers, a few hemophiliacs, transfusion recipients, etc. All others—including Africans—are in the 'unknown risk factor' category. The *real* risk factors, as promulgated by the CDC, are gay sex and dirty needles. This has cast AIDS into a category that transcends the category of 'virus' and lays the disease on the doorstep of 'misbehavior,' which is the way it is often perceived worldwide."

Fettner asserted, "Epidemiologists should report what they find. Period. Not as Jaffe recently did in Belle Glade, predict what they will find, which implies they're looking to prove certain presuppositions. And certainly, epidemiology should not define the social aspects of a disease."

Fettner was more than right that this was "social" epidemiology that had been politically engineered by social insiders about social outsiders. And she was only looking at the tip of an iceberg. It had nothing remotely to do with attentiveness to factual reality. It imposed categories on inconvenient reality and just snipped off any unsightly loose ends that threatened to reveal the truth about the real epidemic.

In the May 5 *Native*, Fettner reported on a journalism conference she attended at the Harvard School of Public Health. There she encountered scientists and reporters who expressed a great deal of contempt for the *Native*. Although Fettner had not covered the ASFV story herself, she was attacked for the *Native*'s coverage of the Teas ASFV hypothesis. Larry Kessler, a Boston AIDS activist, angrily held up a copy of the *Native* after Fettner gave a talk on AIDS reporting and he charged that the *Native* was alarming his "clients." According to Fettner, Harvard AIDS researcher, Jerome Groopman, made a point of announcing to the assembled that ASFV was "not the cause of AIDS because the cause of AIDS is known." *Boston Globe* reporter Judy Forman said that her paper has not reported on Jane Teas's findings of ASFV in AIDS patients because "We decided it was a lot of crap."

Fettner summed up her feelings about the AIDS groupthink that was hardening in cement at that point: "In no other area of science of which I am aware does such an absolute lock of the orthodox philosophy prevail as it does in AIDS. A siege mentality holds fast against opposing views and alternative theories, and those proposing such, regardless of their scientific credentials, are viewed as being part of the lunatic fringe. Not only is this in the remarkably tight scientific circles that have conspired to co-opt research, but also in the reporting on the disease. So restrictive and exclusive has been the formulation of these cadres that no influential person outside these walls has come forward to insist on the legitimacy of alternative ideas. Many privately voice concern over the AIDS 'lockstep,' but fear putting themselves in the position of being branded fringe lunatics—scornfully if they are of marginal reputation, by innuendo if they have an affiliation deemed 'respectable' or susceptible to retaliation."

In the May 26 issue, we published news of what I thought was going to be a real game changer. A story I wrote began, "A potentially important clue in the AIDS epidemic has been discovered by researcher Jane Teas in Belle Glade, Florida. Pigs. Sick pigs. . . . In late April, Teas and [her husband James] Hebert visited Belle Glade to gather ticks, which they intended to have tested to determine if they were carrying African swine fever virus. The spread of AIDS in Belle Glade has been attributed to other factors besides sexual practices and drug use there. Even researchers from the Centers for Disease Control have been quoted as saying that there may be other factors involved in Belle Glade."

I reported, "Teas and Hebert discovered a small pig farm just outside Belle Glade, where they saw between 60 and 80 pigs, some of which were extremely thin and sickly. Are the pigs infected with African swine fever virus? While that remains to be determined by the

U.S. Department of Agriculture, the *Native* has received an unconfirmed report that the pigs in Belle Glade are testing positive for antibodies to HTLV-III."

In the June 9 issue of the paper, I reported on new developments in Belle Glade: "After three years and three months of attempting to bring the connection between AIDS and African swine fever to the world's attention, researcher Dr. Jane Teas may finally have outmaneuvered top officials at the United States Department of Agriculture who have stood in the way of her research. . . . What Dr. Teas found in Belle Glade only substantiated her theory that the solution to the AIDS riddle may be found in part of the world's pig population. She discovered a small dirt-poor farm on which there were 150 pigs. Many of the pigs were sickly, scrawny and dying. The owner of the farm, Ed Wilcox, told Teas that a lot of pigs had died a few months before her visit."

I reported that Teas, along with her husband, James Hebert, and local Belle Glade physician, Mark Whiteside, took blood and tissue samples from the pigs which Jane brought back to Boston and they were subsequently examined by Dr. John Beldekas of Boston University. Teas told me, "The internal organs of several of the slaughtered pigs had lesions that are characteristic of African swine fever."

Beldekas was able to test the pig blood for both ASFV and the so-called AIDS retrovirus, HTLV-III. I reported that Beldekas tested 16 blood samples for ASFV and nine blood samples for HTLV-III. Nearly all of the blood showed positivity by western blot for HTLV-III, and one out of the 16 blood samples tested positive in two different antigen tests for ASFV. Because ASFV is extremely infectious but difficult to detect, if one pig tests positive for the virus, the whole herd is assumed to be infected."

I had notified the USDA of the findings and a veterinarian in Belle Glade was asked to collect pig blood to send to the USDA Plum Island testing facility. I was dismayed that only two samples were being sent to the USDA. I also urged the USDA to take some of the swine blood that Beldekas had found to be positive for HTLV-III and ASFV to see if they could replicate his results. I reported, "On Thursday, May 22, samples arrived at Plum Island. On Tuesday, May 27, the Animal and Plant Health Inspection Service (APHIS) announced to the press that one of the samples tested positive for antibodies to ASFV. It was the same blood sample that tested positive for ASFV antigen in Beldekas's lab."

I notified Jon Nordheimer of the *New York Times* Miami bureau and Keith Schneider of the Washington bureau and both subsequently wrote stories on the ASFV development for the *Times*. APHIS was caught playing games when one APHIS official implied that he would have been nervous about ASFV if the Belle Glade pigs had shown signs of diarrhea, and maintained that the pigs *did not*. A Belle Glade veterinarian, however, told the *Times* that the sick pigs *did have diarrhea*. In addition, Teas and Beldekas, as well as Whiteside, had told me that they had observed that some of the pigs had bloody diarrhea when they had visited the Belle Glade farm—often a telltale sign of African swine fever.

In that same issue, we published a document which I think historians may someday call the smoking gun of the ASFV-AIDS hypothesis. Anne-Christine d'Adesky, who had previously written about the AIDS situation in Haiti, was given a three-inch file of documents on Haiti by a political activist. She reported that among the documents she "came across a memo written to officials at the Haitian Ministry of Agriculture in Damien (outside Port-au-Prince), regarding their participation in the national African swine fever eradication program begun in late 1979. . . . In the memo members of the rural Haitian district of Desforges questioned the plan to kill Haitian pigs and stated that a high number of human deaths from a mysterious fever posed a more immediate threat to their communities. The letter confirms earlier press reports that the Duvalier government ignored information regarding a link between African swine fever and AIDS, [which] developed in the region at the same time."

New York Native published a photocopy of the explosive memo which was sent from several Haitian community councils to the Haitian Minister of Agriculture. The memo began, "Desforges is located 10 km east of the township of Bombardopolis. In the area it rains approximately one month a year, rarely two months. From September to the beginning of the month of February, we have buried three (3) persons every day, all victims of a fever which still persists in the community."

The memo complained that the people in that area of Haiti relied on pigs for financial support. The memo also noted that pigs "allow us to send our children to school, to buy food . . . when hunger sets in." The councils were concerned about "a rumor that all our pigs must be killed before the beginning of March." The councils asked that only pigs that appeared to be sick would be exterminated, something that ran counter to the USDA recommendation that all the Haitian pigs had to be presumed infected or susceptible and therefore had to be killed. The most disturbing and perhaps revealing part of the memo said, "From September to date we have been burying people not pigs, we wonder whether there will be a plan to kill the sick people also. We would like to know what we will live off of when all the pigs have been killed?"

While the memo reflected desperation about how they would survive without the pigs, it also might constitute some kind of inadvertent basic epidemiology indicating that ASFV may have crossed the zoonotic threshold and might have become a human infection. Had officials identified ASFV as the cause of the 1979 deaths mentioned in the Haitian memo, Jane Teas might not have had to fight a losing battle with the USDA and the CDC for over half a decade in a battle to show the AIDS-ASFV connection. The question for forensic historians of the epidemic will be whether those Haitian deaths were the real beginning of the AIDS epidemic in the Western Hemisphere.

On June 23, Robert Gallo was back on the cover of *New York Native*. The headline was "Science's Greatest Living Performer" and the piece provided more evidence that Gallo is one of science's most amazing pathological liars. Ann Giudici Fettner interviewed scientists who worked with Gallo but were afraid to be identified. She wrote, "As you read the following, the result of speaking with several scientists involved with AIDS research at the National Institutes of Health (NIH), it will become apparent why going against the power base is professionally and politically dangerous." About the ongoing battle over who had discovered the so-called AIDS virus, Montagnier or Gallo, she wrote, "Behind the scenes the whole business has generated some extremely hard feelings among the researchers and others involved. What appears in the medical journals for instance, would seem to be merely results of research. Research is reported on, of course, but underlying the selection of data is what seems to be a granite-like agenda to distort the realities of the epidemic into a single theory which increasingly does not hold water. It's as if there are two disparate versions of the disease. One is a research version, the other a clinical version, and the two often have little relationship. Much of this started when the virus was misclassified as belonging to the human T-cell leukemia virus family."

Fettner quoted one anonymous source as saying, "The story is clear to anyone who looks at it rationally. Montagnier—as stupid as he is, and he's a petty little man—the only reason he's still alive today is because Gallo kept him alive. Montagnier discovered a unique virus, but he didn't have the guts to characterize it as his own. He wanted Gallo to hold his hand. So he sent the virus to Gallo twice. First of all, Gallo didn't get it. Then the French produced a bill of lading showing that [Gallo's assistant] Popovic in his lab signed for it. So that's lie number one. Lie number two is that he couldn't get it to grow. That lie has been exposed because of the electron micrograph." (An electron micrograph is a picture of an organism taken through a microscope.)

The source also insisted to Fettner that Gallo calling the French virus a form of "HTLV" was just a ploy to get credit for the discovery. The source also told Fettner, "Now the lie is that he got it to grow but [Gallo argued that] it didn't grow very well. The fact that the sequences are unique proves that's also a lie. They were guilty of intellectual arrogance. They thought since [Montagnier's] virus grew the best—though they had 40 others—they'd just use it; the world would never know the difference."

Fettner also documented the corrupt, authoritarian mess that professional scientific publishing was turning into during the epidemic. She wrote, "One of the major complaints heard from numerous scientists not part of the 'old-boy' network between NIH/NCI/Harvard is the impossibility of getting anything that relates to AIDS published by *Science*. Gallo is routinely called upon to review such papers, and a negative response from him evidently dooms the chance of publication. By the same token, papers from coevals, despite pertinent criticism from reviewers, are slid right through. It is unfortunate that examples of this told to me are from those who would put themselves in jeopardy if the specific cases in point were detailed."

Fettner was one of the first journalists to warn the world about the dangerous power of Robert Gallo. Just as importantly, she was also onto the moral culpability of the rest of the apathetic and morally insensitive scientific community that just let Gallo go his merry way. She concluded her piece noting, "Other scientists laugh when asked about Gallo's patent miscategorizing HTLV-III in the wrong family. Is that funny? I don't think so. Many are defensive when the subject of Montagnier's virus comes up . . . . Meanwhile, millions of lives are at stake as Gallo continues to play games." A middle-aged heterosexual woman with children, Ann Giudici Fettner was not particularly sensitive to the dynamics of heterosexism that may have lurked beneath nervous laughter of the scientists, but she deserves a great deal of credit for noticing that something was seriously out of whack in the scientific community as a whole. Fettner didn't live long enough to see just how many lives Gallo's antics would ultimately cost, but her reporting certainly contributed to a growing awareness that we were entering a period of totalitarian and abnormal science.

On July 22, Phil Donahue hosted a panel of guests on his talk show that discussed the topic of AIDS in the workplace. Near the end of the show, inspired by all the stories about AIDS and African swine fever (and showing the impact the *Native* had on the issue), he asked, "What about pork?" Dr. Mathilde Krim, who was one of the panelists, told Donahue that the involvement of pork and African swine fever virus in AIDS was an outlandish theory that was being investigated. I wrote an open letter to Donahue about the show in our August 4 issue: "I wish that Dr. Krim had given you an answer that was more thorough and more honest about her feelings about this theory, with which you are obviously familiar. I sat in a room with Dr. Krim a few months ago while she listened to a presentation of data on African swine fever, given by Drs. Jane Teas and John Beldekas. It is my understanding that Dr. Krim encouraged Beldekas and Teas to make the long presentation to her board, and she also urged them to apply for a grant from her foundation to continue their research. Shortly after the presentation, Dr. Krim sent a letter to Beldekas encouraging him to continue his work. I was under the impression that Dr. Krim had become quite fascinated by the swine fever theory."

I also told Donahue in that letter, "I would like to encourage you to do a show on AIDS and African swine fever virus. You should also invite the woman who has fought the federal government for over three years in her attempts to research the connection between AIDS and African swine fever. You should also invite Dr. John Beldekas, who found evidence of swine fever infection in AIDS patients, and HTLV-III antibodies in sick pigs in Belle Glade. You should also invite Dr. William Hess and Dr. Richard Wardley, two of the experts on African swine fever who have publicly stated that more research needs to be done."

I also wrote, "You should also invite Dr. James Mason, the director of the Centers for Disease Control, and his sidekick, Dr. James Curran, to defend the actions of the CDC. Having encountered both of these characters on several occasions, I can tell you that your show will be quite entertaining. Maybe you could get Jim Curran to say that he didn't want to explore swine fever because he was afraid of hurting the pork industry. I predict that Mason will mistakenly say 'swine flu' several times as he did in an interview with me. . . . Over the last three years, the government has repeatedly tried to sweep questions about African swine fever and AIDS under the carpet. The CDC and the White House are playing games with the lives of all Americans."

In the same issue, Ann Giudici Fettner wrote about an interesting phone call she had received: "Several weeks ago, Dr. Robert C. Gallo of the National Cancer Institute (NCI), called me early on a Saturday morning to ask, in effect, why I was on his case so hard. The Office of Cancer Communication at the National Institutes of Health (NIH) had told him that my article in [New York Native] was 'the worst thing anyone could have written about him.' Gallo claimed that there were 'some facts' in the article, but that some of it was 'just crap.' He complained about my use of anonymous sources."

Not surprisingly, given his modus operandi, Gallo agreed to be interviewed by Fettner and she met him for several hours a week later in his office at NCI. In the interview, he protested to Fettner that he had no power over who gets grants in research. He told her, "I haven't reviewed a single AIDS grant in my life." He also told her that he made no money from the so-called AIDS test beyond "an inventor's prize of $2,000." He argued that he had all the money he needed and was set because he would inherit money from his successful father. Fettner asked him about rumors he was leaving NIH and he said that his future was up in the air, but that he didn't want "to leave in the middle of the vaccine attempt." (We know how that turned out.) He told Fettner that he didn't think any cofactor was necessary for his retrovirus to cause AIDS. He also insisted that the main lesion in AIDS was "definitely the T-4. Anyone who's studied this can dismiss the T-4 lesion. It's fantastically important. . . . Right now, the field accepts the notion that the infections and cancers arise from immune suppression due to the lack of the central cell of the immune system. The T-4 cell." (And that turned out to be a fantastically simpleminded and wrong. The myopic T-4 paradigm was the big mistake or big fib at the very heart of the bogus science and epidemiology of the epidemic).

In the August 18 issue of *New York Native*, Fettner penned a piece calling for a congressional investigation of the CDC. She wrote, "The Centers for Disease Control AIDS reports and activities are increasingly viewed by impartial researchers with disbelief and anger. Some assign various of the CDC's actions and reports to mere incompetence; others express the view that there may be an agenda to deprive the National Institutes of Health (NIH) of its autonomy; yet others see the CDC as an instrument for helping the Reagan administration to cut expenditures for all health-related measures. In other words, both the CDC's motives and the quality of their science are at issue."

Fettner complained that the CDC was out of touch with the real nature of the epidemic, but, it had "successfully positioned itself as the ultimate authority on AIDS." She argued, "Without question, from the first, political influences have been allowed to intrude on the management of this grave, international health crisis. Having positioned itself as the central authority on AIDS and, given the antagonism they continue to engender between themselves and the scientific community, the activities of the CDC demand outside peer review as well as examination by a select Congressional committee." Fettner quoted Dr. Peter Skrabanek of the University of Dublin as saying, "When epidemiologists begin advising governments" they "declare themselves as agents of social control." (Fettner was onto something far more monstrous than even she, with her sensitive political antennae, recognized.) She wrote that when epidemiologists "choose to become such agents, they leave the sanctified halls of science and enter an arena in which performance and influence are open to examination. The CDC is long overdue for just such an examination. It's time the CDC was called to account. We've had enough of their twisting the epidemic into their own design, whether to cover their erroneous assessments or following an agenda from Washington." Fettner, like most of us back then, didn't realize that the CDC was just getting started.

Fettner also noted, "We have been treated to the CDC's determination to hide black Belle Glade's undoing by AIDS, their lies or incompetence about testing African swine fever-positive sera. I don't know who's ultimately responsible for it and may never know, but I do know it's time to take this disease out of their hands, to get them away from the microphones and reporters. It's also time for a panel of clinical scientists—not enumerators—to decide what is and isn't AIDS. . . . Why are the major researchers standing back and letting the CDC adjudicate at what point one can be diagnosed as having AIDS?"

Fettner once again attacked the top AIDS researcher: "James Curran, head of the CDC's AIDS task force, stood in front of a world audience in Paris and made five-year predictions for the spread of AIDS—based on what? After his plenary session performance, those who know how the epidemiology is being done, and who increasingly despise the CDC's manipulations, came away furious. . . . Does the CDC have information they aren't revealing? In the context of their record for large-scale, long-term predictions, the ones for AIDS have been about as accurate as those of the loonies who periodically appear with signs announcing 'the end of the world is today.' Fettner was onto one of the key aspects of what would turn out to be the CDC's shady way of framing the disease: "The CDC's continually shifting gospel-truth currently asserts that hardly anyone—'fewer than 100'—have survived what the epidemiologists have defined as the 39-month 'natural history,' [of AIDS] but there are probably hundreds who have and do survive. Is it fair to assume that many of these survivors stay away from CDC body counting facilities? I think so."

Unfortunately for the gay community, it would become more and more difficult for people to stay away from the incompetent body counting and the tentacles of the CDC's public health agenda.

Fettner's calls for an investigation fell on deaf ears. In retrospect, she was just seeing the first round of the diabolical game when she noted, "The CDC has consistently mischaracterized AIDS." The bottom of the iceberg—chronic fatigue syndrome and other HHV-6-related conditions—were not fully visible yet. Fettner and the gay community were totally unaware that the blind spot of heterosexism was preventing the medical and scientific establishment from seeing the looming catastrophe ahead.

In the September 15 issue, Gallo was back in the news. I reported that I had learned from a source close to Dr. Robert Gallo that his lab had "isolated a new virus from AIDS patients. The new virus is a DNA virus with a strong resemblance to cytomegalovirus. The source speculated that the new virus may actually be African swine fever virus. . . . According to the source close to Gallo, his lab has also isolated the new DNA virus from a new epidemic, described with various names that is occurring around the country. Some have called this epidemic "non-stop flu," while others term it a variant of mononucleosis. One source [even] refers to it as the 'secondary epidemic of AIDS.' " That epidemic, of course, turned out to be so-called chronic fatigue syndrome.

I pointed out that if African swine fever virus "causes both acute AIDS and a chronic flu-like illness in the general population, it would be imitating the same patterns of infection that occur in herds of pigs infected with ASFV."

Curiously, in terms of the case the *Native* had been building in our reporting about the CDC, in the same issue of the paper, we ran a story by Barry Adkins about a Congressional investigation of the CDC: "Senator Lowell Weicker (R-Conn.) dispatched a Congressional staffer to the . . . CDC AIDS unit in Atlanta on September 3 to investigate charges that researchers had been wrongly fired, and that viral studies had been sabotaged. . . ." Weicker had been concerned about a *Miami Herald* report that suggested that researchers at the CDC had been suppressing and sabotaging AIDS experiments.

In the September 29 issue of the *Native*, Adkins reported, "Numerous incidents of purported sabotage directed at viral projects dealing with the causes of AIDS have been discovered by investigators at the Federal Centers for Disease Control (CDC) in Atlanta. Investigators from outside the agency, as well as internal watchdogs, have uncovered several CDC memos which claim that research has been destroyed by an unknown person or persons over the past several months." The article went on to detail numerous incidents in which AIDS experiments were tampered with or sabotaged. Hopefully historians will one day conduct some forensic work to determine what bearing that sabotage might have had on the scientific truths that were concealed by the CDC during the epidemic.

In November, Ann Fettner strayed off the *Native* reservation and wrote a piece about Robert Gallo's discovery of his mysterious new DNA virus for the *Village Voice*. The virus was called "Human B-cell Lymphotropic Virus" or "HBLV." Based on what I had learned from behind-the-scenes conversations, I reported in our November 3 issue, "Gallo has told the *Native* that he could not rule out the possibility that his new virus is African swine fever virus." I also reported, "Discussions with Fettner have indicated that the epidemiology of the new virus suggests that it may be highly contagious and cause ailments such as flu, encephalitis, multiple sclerosis, arthritis, and possibly AIDS." I noted, "In the American population the new virus is behaving the same way that African swine fever behaved in pigs during the last decade. The new virus is the same size as African swine fever virus. The new virus also looks like cytomegalovirus (CMV) a herpesvirus which the Centers for Disease Control at first thought was the cause of AIDS. African swine fever virus has been confused with [porcine] CMV by researchers in the past." I also wrote, "Fettner's report in the *Voice* that HBLV is now widespread in the population is consistent with the behavior of African swine fever virus, which is highly contagious. Fettner reports that 30% of the people around Lake Tahoe are positive for HBLV." Lake Tahoe was the area in which the cluster of what would be called "chronic fatigue syndrome" was first identified.

In the same article, I noted, "If HBLV [which was eventually called HHV-6] is African swine fever virus, then several strains of swine fever may be circulating in the human population. No strain may be strong enough to cause serious disease. But if humans are now infected by African swine fever virus, the multiple exposures to different strains of the virus could result in serious health problems which in pigs include dermatitis, lymphadenitis, hyperplasia of the lymph nodes, enlarged spleen, hemorrhages, tonsillitis, gastroenteritis, pulmonary edema, interstitial pneumonia, pericarditis and meningo-encephalitis." (The list of pathologies was a foreshadowing of the spectrum of multisystemic dysfunction in chronic fatigue syndrome and HHV-6-related illnesses.)

I also noted in the article that ASFV, like AIDS, was sometimes difficult to recognize because the disease manifestations could be confused with many other diseases. I suggested that the emerging epidemic of Epstein-Barr Virus (EBV), which would eventually be called chronic fatigue syndrome, might "actually be a mild form of African swine fever."

Newsweek had reported, in their October 27 issue, that CFS sufferers "are plagued by low-grade fevers, aching joints, and sometimes a sore throat—but they don't have the flu. They're overwhelmingly exhausted, weak and debilitated—but they don't have AIDS. They're often confused and forgetful—but it isn't Alzheimer's. Many patients feel suicidal, but it isn't clinical depression. They shuttle from doctor to doctor with a variety of symptoms—but it isn't clinical hypochondria." I started to see that the emerging politics of chronic fatigue syndrome were building a biomedical wall of apartheid between CFS and AIDS and I pointed out in my article, "Many if not most, AIDS patients also suffer from reactivated EBV. [Gallo's new DNA virus] HBLV may then turn out to be the cause of viral reactivation and autoimmunity in both AIDS and chronic EBV disease."

In the November 3 issue, I also raised the alarming possibilities that health care workers and AIDS scientists and their families might be at special risk for contracting the newly discovered AIDS-related DNA virus. I reported, "One AIDS researcher told the *Native* that everybody in his lab working on AIDS research has started to show elevated antibodies to Epstein-Barr virus" and I also noted, "One lab research staff has even refused to work with Gallo's new virus. Ironically, every AIDS researcher may have inadvertently been working with HBLV/African swine fever virus for years." (According to a reliable source, there is even a possibility that Gallo brought the virus home to his son, who years later would suffer from chronic fatigue syndrome.)

I also suggested in the article that the new virus would seriously complicate the already treacherous and complex politics of AIDS, especially if Gallo admitted that HBLV was a human adaptation of African swine fever virus. The merging of a human health problem with an animal disease involving a staple of the American diet in a brand new epidemiological narrative was potentially an apocalyptic political and biomedical mess.

Curiously, at the same time, officials in New Jersey were considering halting regular testing of pigs for ASFV in that state. *New York Native* had raised questions about the wisdom of that move and on May 7, 1986, a USDA official, Dr. E.C. Sharman, wrote in a memo, "New Jersey was exploring the possibility of discontinuation of sampling about a year ago. We encouraged them to continue participating at that time. The discontinuation of ASFV sampling if it became known to the gay community may provide ammunition for falsely accusing us of 'hiding the existence of the disease in the country.'" It's amusing that the little *New York Native* was basically being perceived as "the gay community." Would that it were so. And even if true, who knew that the gay community could so easily affect the policies of the USDA?

I also reported, in that same piece, that I had spoken to a clinician in Atlanta who had told me that he had seen cases of the new chronic EBV infection [that turned out to be chronic fatigue syndrome] *at the same time he started seeing AIDS cases.* I noted, "Gallo's new virus HBLV may be the cause of both epidemics. If HBLV is African swine fever virus, the linkage would make a great deal of sense. African swine fever is not [strictly speaking] a sexually transmitted disease, but the outcome of the infection may be tied to the number of exposures, amount of exposure, immune status of the host and the orifice in which the virus is contracted." I also reported, "When I talked to Robert Gallo on Wednesday, October 22, I urged him to resolve the matter of whether HBLV is African swine fever virus as soon as possible. I told him that even the safety of his lab workers was at stake. He told me that the materials which he planned to use to test whether his new virus is African swine fever were from the USDA were not of sufficient quality to make a determination, and that the matter is still unresolved. I urged him to contact the USDA's Director of Animal Health and Inspection Service, Burt Hawkins, to obtain the materials necessary to do a DNA probe—a test which Gallo feels is necessary to determine if HBLV is African swine fever virus. I asked Gallo if he would change the name of his new virus from HBLV to African swine fever virus if it turns out that the viruses are identical. He replied, 'You have an absolute promise that if this is African swine fever virus, the name will be changed instantly.' "

In my December 1 editorial, I commented on a *New York Times* November 7, 1986, editorial which asked, "Is AIDS about to become epidemic among the general public in America, too?" The editorial insisted, "The evidence of breakout is far from conclusive." I wrote, "The problem is that the *Times* remains convinced that HTLV-III is the cause of AIDS. The pattern of HTLV-III infection has been reassuring to the *Times*. . . . Imagine how catastrophically wrong the *Times* might be if HTLV-III is not the cause of AIDS. . . . When the *Times* bases scientific conclusions on data from the CDC, they are using public relations data, not science. HTLV-III has not been shown to be the cause of AIDS. HTLV-III has been declared the cause of AIDS. There is a difference." I asked, "What if AIDS is caused by HBLV, the new virus which Robert Gallo is now comparing with African swine fever virus? First of all, we need new epidemiology. Preliminary reports from Lake Tahoe suggest that 30% or more of the general population is infected with HBLV. If HBLV is the cause of AIDS, then we are in the middle of a major pandemic whereby entire American cities and towns could begin the same source of suffering as cities and towns in Africa. No scientist has yet tried to force HBLV into the category of sexually transmitted viruses, because the pattern of infection is too widespread and appears to be too casual. HBLV may escape the control of the VD moralists at the CDC. Is HBLV to be found in 100% of the blood of people with AIDS? Not yet according to Dr. Gallo. His staff has found it in only 30% of AIDS patients but Dr. Gallo notes that these are early findings, and his assay is still imperfect."

In the editorial I suggested that New York City's Health Commissioner, Dr. Stephen Joseph should "put together a task force to study the relationship between HBLV and AIDS. Among the areas that should be investigated are: 1) What percentage of health care workers are now infected with HBLV? 2) What can be done to prevent health care workers from spreading HBLV to patients in their hospitals? 3) What percentage of AIDS researchers are now infected with HBLV? 4) Is HBLV a virus that is present in any animals that are consumed by humans? 5) Should the Blood Center be screening blood for HBLV?"

In the December 8 issue, I raised questions about the judgment of the man who was quickly becoming the country's de facto AIDS Czar: "Tony Fauci, the young (46-year-old) director of the National Institute of Allergy and Infectious Diseases (NIAID) was profiled by Christine Russell in the November 3, 1986, issue of *The Washington Post*. Young Fauci may be one of the most powerful people in AIDS politics in America." I pointed out that his institute then controlled 60% of the total AIDS budget. I noted, "He came across as an insensitive jerk" when he spoke about AIDS publicly earlier that year. I wrote that Fauci's bedside manner is not as worrisome to me as the fact that he's a man with a hypothesis about AIDS that may be dead wrong, and his own honor may be on the line every time any part of NIAID's budget is spent on AIDS research. The question in my mind is this: Is Tony Fauci an American Lysenko?"

In the 1930s, Trofim Denisovich Lysenko was a Russian scientist who had ideas about agriculture that turned out to be dead wrong. According to *Betrayers of the Truth*, the groundbreaking book on scientific fraud by Nicholas Wade and William Broad, the Russian government threw its complete political and financial support behind Lysenko's crackpot agricultural ideas in 1935. Wade and Broad note, "It was an act of willful desperation. The bureaucrats realized they were not making much progress with the agricultural situation; . . . so the bureaucrats chose a bureaucratic solution, which was to put someone in charge and let him cope with the problem. Unfortunately, the person they chose was Lysenko." In my editorial I asked if "AIDS is a similar situation and does Fauci have the power of a Lysenko? Science in America is an expensive proposition and he who controls funding also controls science. In Russell's profile of Fauci, she notes that one scientist described Fauci's "insistence on keeping his laboratory [as] a potential danger . . . because 'it brings all sorts of suspicion,' however unfounded that his loyalties to his lab might interfere with his duties as an impartial institute director." I also noted that Russell reported that one of Fauci's colleagues said, "There is something in him that has to show people he can do it all." Fauci had at least one prescient colleague. One could say that Fauci came closest to being the epidemic's control freak. Or worse.

In that same issue of the *Native*, we reported that William Buckley retracted his "AIDS tattoo" proposal for HIV positive people after a meeting with representatives of the Gay and Lesbian Alliance Against Defamation. (I'd love to see a film reenactment of *that* meeting.) His proposal first appeared on the March 18, 1986, *New York Times* op-ed page and before that in his nationally syndicated column. He also made the proposal on his PBS television program, *Firing Line.* "Everyone," Buckley wrote, "detected with AIDS should be tattooed in the upper forearm to protect common-needle users, and on the buttocks, to prevent the victimization of other homosexuals."

Serendipitously, in the same issue of *New York Native*, we published an interview with Richard Plant by Allen Ellenzweig about Plant's book, *The Pink Triangle: The Nazi War Against Homosexuals.* Plant had been a friend of Hannah Arendt's and a professor at the New School. We also published a brief excerpt from Plant's book with this chilling passage: ". . . Himmler was not optimistic about the prospects of rehabilitating men suffering from the disease of homosexuality. Perhaps a few hustlers might be salvaged, but he was doubtful about the immoral homosexual majority. Not long after, he would come to believe that the final solution was inevitable for gays as for Jews and other 'contragenics.' He dubbed it 'delousing,' a term favored by other Nazi theoreticians as well." One could say that Himmler was an AIDS epidemiologist before his time.

1987: An Epic Epidemiological Battle

In the January 12 issue of *New York Native,* I wrote about a December 27, 1986, interview in *The Washington Post* with Robert Redfield, a top military doctor involved in AIDS research. I suggested that if the interview was any indication, the gay community was in for a wild new round of scapegoating and repression. Redfield was a proponent of universal testing for HTLV-III (HIV) and he was one of the first people to start directing veiled threats at those who stood in the way of the government's AIDS agenda. According to *The Washington Post* interview conducted by Phil Hilts, Redfield said, "Anyone who tries to persuade people not to get tested 'has the blood of more gay men on his hands.' "

According to Hilts, Redfield issued a major warning to the gay community on HTLV-III (HIV) testing. He told Hilts that not testing and not telling " 'is threatening the health of the whole community. And ultimately it's going to threaten [gays'] freedom. They don't understand it, but a lot of people are going to be angry when they learn that public health authorities of our country have been paralyzed because of this concern about confidentiality. . . .' "

Ironically, after making a threat that would become an all too familiar motif of the epidemic, Redfield urged the gay community to trust people like himself. Hilts reported that Redfield "believes people must summon enough trust to begin more widespread testing for AIDS." Redfield then mouthed words to Hilts that are some of the most haunting of the whole AIDS era: " 'Lots of doctors run away when their patients die. I maybe started to do that a little, because I have been through so many deaths in this epidemic. But I try to make a point of not running away; I want to help them die, and to work the family through it.' "

In the same issue, we reported on measures then being taken by police in Germany that might have pleased Redfield. In the city of Munich the police were keeping files on homosexuals. According to John J. Vischansky, the lists included "the names of customers" who patronized "gay bookstores and sex shops," "patrons identified in raids on gay bars and cruising areas," "the names of people passing by and identified in the vicinity of gay bars at night," "anybody whose papers have been checked in a public restroom or close to one, no matter what the reason," and "known or admitted homosexuals, transvestites and call boys." Vischansky reported, "For years, the German police have publicly, flatly, and officially denied the existence of such lists, which in part date back to the years long before homosexuality was decriminalized in Germany. Nevertheless, just a few weeks ago, a commission set up to review compliance with federal legislation on data privacy stumbled over these lists."

Vischansky also reported, "The president of the Munich police department, Gustav Haring . . . justified the failure to erase these files "because of the danger of AIDS, which is especially widespread among this group of persons. Gay groups have called for Haring's resignation, to no avail. Worse yet, Haring's boss at the time, Peter Gurweiller, had the gall to state, 'The purpose of [the] regulation is to prevent the epidemic from being spread to families and from affecting the totally innocent.' "

In the January 19 issue of the *Native*, I published a letter that I had written to Burt Hawkins, the Administrator of the Animal and Plant Health Inspection Service (APHIS). I noted in the letter that he must have been aware that Dr. Gallo had stated for the record that he could not rule out the possibility that the newly discovered DNA virus, Human B-Cell Lymphotrophic Virus (HBLV) is actually African swine fever virus. I told him I had heard that APHIS was preparing a DNA probe to help determine whether HBLV is ASFV. I expressed my surprise that this was taking so long since ASFV is one of the most lethal viruses known to the USDA. I wrote, "Surely you must realize that if a scientist of Gallo's caliber suggests a possible relationship . . . the matter should be taken very seriously. I assumed that the [possible] presence of ASFV in our country was considered a national emergency, and would be dealt with in a matter of hours, not weeks or months. You have the necessary expertise. By letting this take so long, I think you and your department have let the country down in this matter."

Twenty days after I sent my letter, I received a response from J.K. Atwell, the Deputy Administrator of the USDA Veterinary Services. He wrote, "An approved diagnostic DNA probe for ASFV has not been developed. . . . bacterial plasmids containing ASFV DNA segments have been developed by the Agricultural Research Service at their Plum Island Animal Disease Laboratory that may be of assistance in distinguishing between ASFV and Dr. Robert C. Gallo's newly discovered HBLV. This product has been promised to Dr. Gallo. However, since it is presently located in a restricted laboratory, it must be safety tested before it can be removed from Plum Island. When this testing is completed, this research product will be provided to Dr. Gallo."

In the January 25 issue, we published another angry rant by Larry Kramer in the form of an open letter to Richard Dunne, the head of Gay Men's Health Crisis. The letter, like everything Kramer wrote, was premised on the CDC's epidemiology and virology. The letter began, "The doomsday scenario that many have feared for so long comes closer. Next week 274 people will die from AIDS. Next week 374 more will become infected with the killer virus. In four years at least 270,000 people will have AIDS. Of these, 179,000 will have died. Four million people already are infected. As many as 50% of these millions will die. Two out of three AIDS cases are still happening to gay men."

His letter criticized Dunne and GMHC for not being prepared for what was coming. He urged GMHC to "fight for gay men." The paradigm that Kramer promoted in the letter was the one he pushed throughout the epidemic which tragically meant that he generally got everything exactly backwards. He attacked Dunne for not standing up to "a world filled with heterosexual connivance almost bordering on collusion at the least and conspiracy at the most—ignoring us, treating us like so much offal fit to die in agony while tests, trials, delays, ignorance, inhuman uncaring, lying, ass dragging, characterize the daily activities of just about everyone and everything in sight, particularly the 'appropriate medical journals.' " Kramer wanted a kind of whirling dervish political activity to occur on every front except the one that absolutely mattered the most to the gay community: the AIDS establishment's questionable epidemiology and virology which *really were* replete with what he called "heterosexual connivance." If there is anything more heterosexually conniving and apartheid*ish* in human history than the "HIV causes AIDS and CFS isn't AIDS" paradigm, I don't know what it is.

Kramer also wrote, "I do not *care* what the *New England Journal of Medicine* reports about AIDS; or *Science* or *The Lancet* or the *Journal of the American Medical Association*. From the very beginning of this epidemic, they have shown scant concern for us, for our rights, for our continued health survival on this planet."

Not caring what was being reported about AIDS in the world's leading medical journals, was a very strange way of being attentive to what was happening to the gay community. Like it or not, the fate of the gay community and the epidemic was being negotiated in these very journals. The problem wasn't the "scant concern." Au contraire. The problem was that garbage-in-garbage-out epidemiology and its consequential misguided virology were being published on a nonstop basis, and Kramer, because he was blind to the fact that the epidemiological fundamentals were replete with "heterosexual connivance almost bordering on collusion," ended up being a fraud enabler and a hapless cheerleader for the underlying deceit and self-deceit of the epidemic. It is ironic that he screamed at Dunne in his letter, "How dare you be so trusting and naïve—you who are head of Gay Men's Health Crisis?" This is one of the great pot-meets-kettle moments in the Kramer legacy. He was not the first person in history to excel at what could be called the politics of the tantrum which were a poor substitute for well-informed and savvy political judgment—and due diligence. Perhaps young minority communities with no political compass are particularly susceptible to the kind of outrageous narcissistic and delusional performance art posing as canny activism that Kramer offered.

In Kramer's letter, he accused GMHC of becoming fat and rich, a "bastion of conservatism" an organization that would no longer "fight for the living." GMHC had become a "funeral home," "cowardly." One of the more darkly ironic things he said to Dunne in his letter was, "You and your huge assortment of caretakers perform miraculous tasks helping the dying to die." But what he wanted GMHC to do was to "fight" for the living. He wanted them to "use their strength to confront our enemies, to make them help us. This is what political strength is about. It is all." Actually, in the context of the epidemic, real political strength would have been forcing the government to tell the entire inconvenient truth about what was really going on. Or just daring to find out the truth for ourselves.

The point Kramer was missing was the war he didn't even know the gay community really had to fight: an epic epidemiological battle. Like all the woodenheaded collaborators of the epidemic, Kramer called for more "education." Insofar as Kramer was urging GMHC to "fight for the education of everyone," he was basically calling for GMHC to fight for more *HIV propaganda* bearing the CDC's hardwired antigay epidemiology. He was inadvertently calling for more shovels to dig gay graves.

Kramer's call for GMHC to fight for more drug trials was of course based on the premise that the CDC had gotten the virology of AIDS *right*. That premise ended up getting a lot of people poisoned thanks to the clueless activists who had been urged to "fight" a battle they couldn't even fully comprehend. AZT was the great hope at that time and not yet perceived to be the iatrogenocidal disaster that it actually was. Kramer wrote in his letter to Dunne, "It is now reported that AZT is going to cost each patient $5,000 a year when it becomes available. What are you doing to confront this abhorrent future, in which few patients will be able to afford the very drug that might save them?" Unfortunately, it would turn out that the cost was not the biggest problem with AZT. Its high cost may actually have *saved* some lives. Complaining about the cost or AZT turned out to be like complaining about the high cost of a train ticket to Auschwitz.

In retrospect, it is amusing to note that at this point in the epidemic, Kramer still admired what we were doing in the pages of *New York Native*. He chided Dunne and GMHC, writing, "Why do you not ride herd on research rather than leaving it to others (such as the *Native*) to cry out in alarm when false trails are championed and legitimate avenues are ignored?" Alas, Kramer followed the *Native* only so far down those avenues.

In more of the Kramer style of irony, he wrote that Dunne and GMHC "continue to deny the political realities of this epidemic. There is nothing in the whole AIDS mess that is not political. How can you continue to deny this fact and assert that your role must remain unpolitical?"

And even more ironically, in terms of Kramer's own petulant intolerance for differing opinions, he wrote, "You have shut out every dissenting voice you have effectively cut yourselves off from much of the gay community. If anyone doesn't agree with you they are ignored."

Near the end of his letter, Kramer inadvertently nailed not only the problem with GMHC but also the problem with Larry Kramer: "We are all exceptionally tired. We are all AIDSed out. In our exhaustion. Let Someone Else Do It. In our exhaustion, we foster our continued ignorance; we don't keep up with what is going on; we don't want to know; we don't read the *Native*; we don't read every article on AIDS. In this ignorance and exhaustion is our destruction." These words belong on the AIDS community's collective tombstone—and Larry Kramer's. Looking back at the Kramer legacy, one always has to ask the question, "Did this guy ever listen to anything he himself was saying?" Kramer would eventually lead the gay community in a formal huffy exodus from the *Native*, unable to face the uncompromising truths that the *Native* kept publishing until its demise at the beginning of 1997.

A story about a magazine survey of doctors, which we ran in the February 2 issue, presented a stark warning to the gay community about the attitudes it could face from the medical community throughout the epidemic. The survey had been published in the January issue of *MD Magazine*. According to the poll, seventy-eight percent of the respondents favored contact tracing of high risk (guess who?) patients followed by tracing and testing all sexual partners. Thirty-five percent favored testing food handlers and most disturbingly, 28 percent favored some form of quarantine. These were the people who would, in their medical practices, activate and promote the public health agenda that followed logically and inexorably from the CDC's us-versus-them epidemiology.

In the February 9 issue, we published several pages of letters from GMHC's workers and supporters in defense of the organization that Larry Kramer had attacked as being run by a bunch of apolitical sissies. In retrospect, my favorite letter, from a person named Gordon Grant, was also the briefest: "Regarding Ms.(sic) Kramer's open letter to GMHC . . . sissies—feh! You old bitchy queen."

We published a long piece on the Tuskegee Syphilis Experiment by Martin Levine in the February 16 issue. The disturbing article began, "They say we have bad blood. Nearly forty years ago they told some black men that they had bad blood." Levine then recounted the details of the forty-year experiment in which public health authorities conducted a study that monitored the effects of untreated syphilis in poor black sharecroppers in the South. Levine discussed James Jones's classic account of the experiment, *Bad Blood*. At the end of the article Levine voiced the concerns he felt about the warnings the Tuskegee Syphilis Experiment had for the gay community: "In both Tuskegee and AIDS the socially franchised studied the socially disenfranchised. White doctors experimented upon illiterate black men. Heterosexual researchers explore a disease which usually strikes gay men, as well as Haitians, intravenous drug users, and hemophiliacs." He pointed out, "While there are a few gays involved in the Centers for Disease

Control's work on AIDS, the overwhelming majority of the staff is straight. Consider the composition of the AIDS Activity's Group's full-time personnel. Those working exclusively at headquarters number ten—seven doctors, two public health professionals, and one research sociologist. All of them are straight; one is an orthodox Jew and another is a deacon in his church."

Surprisingly, even after writing a book like *Bad Blood*, James Jones still didn't see much for gays to automatically worry about. Levine wrote, "What do these similarities [between the Tuskegee Syphilis Experiment and AIDS] mean? After listing them for the author of Bad *Blood*, I asked what implications he thought Tuskegee had for us. Dr. Jones replied, "The Centers for Disease Control has done a lot that is wrong, a lot that is heroic. The fact that they were responsible for the Tuskegee experiment does not automatically mean they will exploit a minority group. The information in *Bad Blood* needs to be shared and raised as a note of caution. You have every right to be cautious, but don't fear conspiracy until the hard evidence is in."

Levin reported, "In the last few weeks I have discussed Tuskegee with gay people working on AIDS across the country. All reacted deeply to Tuskegee's unethical nature, racist overtones, and methodological flaws. All felt it had significant implications for AIDS. Many of the people I spoke to are not in a position to be quoted publicly. Two were most concerned about ethics. They wondered if the researchers were again violating human experimentation regulations. 'The researchers are gathering gay men's names, addresses, and sexual histories. The public disclosure of this information could potentially harm those men. I see no safeguards for protecting the men's anonymity,' said a person working with AIDS victims in San Francisco. This individual further commented upon the failure of some researchers to get informed consent from the men. Another worried about the possible danger in the Centers for Disease Control's case studies. 'They are going around the country collecting names and addresses of gay men. Can we trust them not to use the lists in harmful ways? What are they doing with it?' "

Levin also reported, "Others wondered if the research had homophobic overtones. Racist science prompted the Tuskegee experiment. It was thought that the innate characteristics of blacks made them sexually promiscuous. 'This notion has become the foundation for all the Centers for Disease Control's studies. From the onset, they theorized that if AIDS hit gay men, it had to be because they were promiscuous,' said a person closely connected to the [CDC]."

Most presciently, Dr. Stephen Murray, a San Francisco based sociologist, told Levine, " 'If Tuskegee was such poor science, why not AIDS? . . . All they have done is taken a group of sick people and seen what they have. It is nothing more than the correlations based on a sample of the sick, and all while the relationship may be caused by a third factor. And from this they build an infectious agent theory, and panic the public into believing our blood is diseased. It's a medical counterrevolution—from the mental hospitals to the quarantine.' "

On March 9, we published a piece by John Lauritsen in which he reviewed a report on AIDS prepared by a committee sponsored by the National Academy of Sciences and The Institute of Medicine. Lauritsen noted, "This report was intended to inform an appropriate national response to the various problems arising from AIDS . . . . The resultant report—nearly 400 pages of highly condensed and often technical material—reflects an enormous amount of intellectual effort. It is an impressive performance in every respect save one: the logic of its underlying premises."

Lauritsen criticized the report's assumption, from its very first page, that HIV without any qualifications was the cause of AIDS. He noted that at one point in the report "reference is made to 'HIV *and its unambiguous identification as the AIDS virus*' which is rhetorical overkill." He argued, "In fact HIV has consistently failed to fulfill even a single one of Koch's postulates, the series of tests which medical science has traditionally required a microbe to pass before it can be considered the cause of a particular disease." Lauritsen had found his way into the opposite world of abnormal science.

One of the best examples of the lack of scientific standards operating in the field of AIDS research is the fact that, as Lauritsen points out, nowhere in the report "is convincing evidence presented which could establish HIV as the cause of AIDS; at the same time, evidence is occasionally cited which would suggest either HIV is not the cause of AIDS, or that it plays a causal role only in conjunction with other, potent cofactors." He pointed out the epidemiological embarrassment in the report which "acknowledges that it is impossible to isolate HIV from many AIDS patients and that some AIDS patients show no evidence of ever having been infected with the virus. (That is to say, they are negative for HIV itself, as well as for HIV antibodies.)"

Lauritsen criticized the report for suggesting that HIV was

responsible for the depletion of T4-cells when in fact "HIV appears to infect very few T4-cells." And "in AIDS patients, the immunological functioning of all T-cells is severely compromised. The cells are sick regardless of whether or not they are 'infected' (nearly all of them are not) and regardless of what the T-cell ratio may happen to be." Lauritsen wrote, "It is mysterious that the authors do not entertain the possibility that something other than HIV is responsible for weakening all of the T-cells." He was concerned that recreational drugs were responsible and that their role was completely ignored by the report.

Lauritsen took issue with the report's assumption that IV drug users were developing AIDS because they shared needles, noting that it wasn't certain if all those affected had even shared needles, and perhaps more importantly, the fact that health care workers were not getting AIDS from needlestick injuries involving AIDS patients made the whole HIV theory doubtful.

In his piece, Lauritsen asserted, "Before the 'AIDS virus' bandwagon really got under way, AIDS was understood as a condition. . . . Now that HIV ideology has achieved almost total hegemony, AIDS has come to be conceptualized as a disease: 'HIV infection.' " He took issue with "the equation of AIDS with HIV" arguing, "A not-inconsiderable proportion of AIDS patients show no evidence of ever having been infected with HIV" and "hundreds of thousands of people are estimated to be HIV seropositive, and yet the vast majority of them are not sick in any way."

Lauritsen argued that the CDC acted in a Procrustean manner in the way they manipulated their definition of AIDS. If a case of AIDS had no evidence of HIV, it was not considered AIDS, but according to Lauritsen, "At the same time, the CDC is sufficiently flexible that if confronted with an AIDS case with negative tests for both virus and antibodies, it can also declare *on faith* that the patient is infected with HIV, even though there is no evidence that he is." Lauritsen was floored by the crazy logic and asserted, "May it be recorded in the annals of science that the CDC succeeded linguistically in establishing HIV as the cause of AIDS, even though the virus never succeeded in fulfilling even one of Koch's postulates."

Lauritsen was troubled by the predictions the committee made in the report about how many of the seropositive would develop AIDS and how large the epidemic would become in America. He was also alarmed that their recommendations for future spending and research revolved around the assumption that HIV was the true cause.

Lauritsen argued, "We need to know the characteristics of people with AIDS. As it is now, we know almost nothing about the gay men with AIDS other than the 'homosexual/bisexual' label that has been slapped on them." He described the original epidemiology of AIDS done by the CDC as being out of date and incompetent.

Lauritsen was onto the fact that the whole affair was political: "The patient characteristics statistics, which the CDC periodically releases to the media, have been incomplete and misleading. We have no idea, for example, what percentage of the total AIDS cases are Haitians; the CDC described, for political reasons, that Haitians should disappear as a 'risk group,' and disappear they did." Unfortunately gay men did not have the political clout to make themselves disappear from the CDC's skewed epidemiology.

Lauritsen excoriated the report for ignoring the role of cofactors like recreational drugs, the centerpiece of his personal AIDS theory. He was concerned that an educational campaign to stop the transmission of HIV, the questionable official cause of AIDS, ignored the toll that recreational drugs *by themselves* would continue to have in destroying the immune systems of those who would eventually be diagnosed with AIDS.

Ominously, Lauritsen wrote that while the report suggested, "Coercive measures would not be effective in altering the course of the epidemic" they "are by no means ruled out completely. Indeed, having painted the picture of a *killer virus* on the loose, of more than a quarter of a million AIDS cases in the U.S. alone in the next four years, the committee might have been more consistent had they called for draconian measures to control the spread of infection." It was another symptom of the bizarre logic of abnormal science.

Lauritsen came to a Barbara Tuchmanesque conclusion about the whole report, noting that it "illustrates once again that group intelligence is below individual intelligence—that even a committee composed of brilliant individuals, as this one appears to have been, is capable of monumental folly. In sum, this is a well-intentioned book which has a great potential for harm."

In the same issue of *New York Native,* the possibility of coercion got all too real in a story by Bill Bahlman about a resolution that was introduced in the New York City Council by Council member Joseph Lisa. His resolution "would allow forced testing for antibodies, to HIV (the so-called AIDS virus), contact tracing of sexual partners of those who test positive, as well as possible quarantine for those who are

HIV-antibody positive, those with AIDS-related complex, and persons with AIDS (PWAs)." Interestingly, according to Bahlman, "Only one witness testified in favor of the resolutions, Dr. Robert Redfield, former head of Walter Reed Army Medical Center."

Topping everything off in that issue, Mike Salinas reported that the Indian government had begun deporting foreign students who tested positive for antibodies to HIV.

In the March 16 issue, we published a long account, written by Darrell Yates Rist, about a two-day forum held by the CDC on "The Role of AIDS Virus Antibody Testing in the Prevention and Control of AIDS." The more appropriate title would have been "The Role of AIDS Virus Antibody Testing in the Persecution and Control of the Gay Community and Others." Rist reported that the CDC director, the devout Mormon, James O. Mason, opened the conference saying, "In coming together these two days we have one purpose in mind: to define a common enemy. The enemy is not me, it is not public health, it is not the people who have expressed interest in civil liberties." (Well, he got one out of three right.) Mason spoke the language of inexorable public health logic: "In the face of a deadly virus, we are determining now what is best for the health of the nation, not what makes people happy." This is the kind of "health of the nation" rhetoric that would also have wowed the perpetrators of the hybrid of medicine and politics that was the Third Reich.

Rist reported on the categories of testing Mason described that were up for debate which ranged from strictly voluntary to mandatory. Rist questioned the CDC's sudden agnosticism on the testing issue, pointing out, "This was a very different tale from the one that had hit the press in early February when according to the *New York Times* (among a host of other papers), the CDC was urging mandatory tests for hospital admissions, pregnant women, patients at STD clinics, and applicants for marriage licenses."

In retrospect, Rist's sociological description of the CDC meeting is quite revealing: "This is a new community of purpose born of AIDS, public health, and civil liberties, which confounds the sexual orientation lines—the ever-more-easy assimilation that many gays will argue is the goal of fighting for gay rights. And many of the lesbians and gays at the conference in Atlanta, it would seem, find themselves more comfortable here than they ever did among the strict devotees of the 'movement.' " One could say that Rist had taken an inadvertent

Polaroid snapshot of the gay community's incipient collaboration in its own self-destruction. To borrow from Arendt, they were essentially assimilating to the biomedical heterosexism of the fraudulent "HIV is AIDS" and "chronic fatigue syndrome is not AIDS" paradigms.

One of the more memorable images in Rist's article on the CDC forum was provided by a member of a small group (only 5 people) named the Lavender Hill Mob, a so-called radical gay group that basically was there to show rage and to yell that people should be angry and yelling. Rist reported that Lavender Hill Mob member Michael Petrelis, who was dressed in "faux concentration camp garb with a pink triangle and an ID number stitched to the pocket on his shirt," asked Mason if he would "take the test and announce your antibody status to the press?" Petrelis was not onto the real game. That was *exactly* the kind of thing the CDC wanted to happen in every quarter of American society. (Flash forward to the Obama years during which it seems like Obama and his wife turned publicly taking HIV tests into public health agitprop.) Rist wrote that in response, "Mason smiled, as though he'd been confronted not so much by an evil devil as a silly one, and said, 'We're tryin' to find a way to save you guys' lives,' and punched the air towards Petrelis's arm paternally."

Rist noted that all the panels during the forum failed to do one basic thing: question the epidemiology and virology. He wrote, "No one questioned whether or not this virus, HIV, is the cause of AIDS or merely a cofactor or simply a marker. No one questioned whether or not this antibody test for HIV is accurate. . . . No one questioned *testing* (except for the [Lavender Hill] Mob, and then not coherently.) It was, everybody seemed to think, a boon to the public health . . . ."

Rist reported that, "The ACLU [American Civil Liberties Union] acquiesced perfunctorily to the good of the antibody tests." (Generally speaking, the ACLU was good for nothing but acquiescing throughout the epidemic.)

Rist also reported that 19 AIDS advisory and service organizations signed a "consensus statement" (which ultimately helped seal the fate of the gay community). It called for testing that was anonymous "coupled with in-depth counseling." "Counseling" of course became another working euphemism for propaganda during the epidemic.

One of the absurdly self-defeating things the gay community did throughout the epidemic was to constantly—in an insipid, abject manner—call for more "education." Had the call been for "re-education" it would have been on the money. When the professional gays and AIDS activists weren't calling for education, they were calling for the funding of "prevention" which was basically a call for more "education." They turned the gay community into one big AIDS re-education camp.

Rist caught the degree to which gays were politically deprived of a seat at the table at this very political forum. One gay leader complained to him, "Gay groups weren't included in the panels (though individually, openly gay people were) . . ." Bizarrely, Urvashi Vaid, of NGLTF told Rist, "Being visible as the NGLTF or GMHC or whoever is not always the route to take." You could call it the gay politics of self-imposed invisibility, a novel form of closeted politics. Gay leader Tim Sweeney manifested these absurd politics when he told Rist, "The way to kill mandatory testing is to go for the public health angle, not civil liberties. The people who need to be convinced don't want to hear from gay organizations." The politically more astute gay leader, Ben Shatz, saw what was really happening and told Rist, "I think it sets a precedent for further exclusion. . . . When we lose visibility we lose power."

One of the more bizarre political developments in the epidemic was the establishment of the opposite world meme that discrimination against the HIV positive was bad because it discouraged HIV testing—a premise that had several diabolical homophobic layers. Robert Redfield, the Army doctor who attended the forum, represented the craziness of the meme beautifully, when according to Rist, he said, "As long as there's a perception of discrimination, it interferes with routine testing to help control the epidemic. We must support the kind of anti-discrimination measures talked about today." Anti-discrimination was really a Trojan horse for medical testing and the incorporation of gays into a Brave New Epidemiological Paradigm. Right before one's eyes one could see the morphing of the fight against discrimination directed towards gays becoming the fight against discrimination toward the HIV positive, which turned the paradigm of gay liberation upside down and inside out. Invisibly it insidiously supported the fraudulent presumption that HIV was the cause of AIDS, while subsuming the fight for gay civil liberties under the Orwellian logic and stigma of public health measures. Throughout the epidemic, gay rights would be supported as a way of fighting AIDS, creating an unprecedented toxic hybrid of self-defeating politics and fraud-based medicine for the gay community.

In the same issue, we published a story about an historic meeting between the Gay and Lesbian Alliance Against Defamation and the editors of the *New York Times*: "The discussion ranged from the GLAAD claims of *Times* undercoverage of gay events and the political implications of AIDS, to the *Times* refusal to use the word 'gay' except in direct quotation." The world's leading newspaper, the one that would be the first and last word on AIDS, always giving the rest of the media its marching orders, couldn't even call gays "gay." (It was amazing how quickly the supposedly very liberal *New York Times* adopted the pernicious and breathtakingly stupid trend of using the insulting word "queer" less than a decade after that meeting. More on that later.)

In the June 15 issue, Mike Salinas covered an ACT UP demonstration that took place across from the White House. According to Salinas, the protestors were pressing for five initiatives that included a "Manhattan Project" on AIDS, "a guarantee of confidentiality between doctor and patient," and "a national AIDS policy to prohibit discrimination against persons infected with HIV." This was yet another Potemkin protest that in essence supported the government's HIV ideology and propaganda.

Salinas reported, "The Reagan administration was still smarting from what it considered to be the bad manners of the dying and their friends, who had booed the president during his speech, the night before, at a fundraising dinner for the American Foundation for AIDS Research (amfAR). During that speech (his first attempt to explain his position on the epidemic since he assumed the presidency), Reagan pledged his support for what he called 'routine testing.' Although it remains unclear exactly what Reagan meant by that, he did outline his hopes that couples seeking marriage licenses, Federal prisoners, and aliens applying for American residence would be subject to blood tests to determine the possible presence of antibodies to HIV, the so-called 'AIDS virus.' "

Salinas noted, "Those who heard the President's speech were clearly shocked by such an idea—which had already been discussed by health officials and dismissed as unworkable for several reasons—and almost equally dismayed that he had chosen the amfAR dinner as the forum to announce it. A chorus of boos and hisses greeted the President's proposal, leaving him 'visibly shaken,' according to sources. Actress Elizabeth Taylor, chairperson of The American Foundation for AIDS Research, was 'rattled' by the heckling said the *New York Post*, and [Surgeon General] Koop was quoted as saying he was 'embarrassed' by it."

Meanwhile, ACT UP protestors in Washington D.C.'s Lafayette Park were met by police who were wearing yellow latex gloves. Salinas reported that the "offended crowd shouted 'Take off the gloves' furiously to no avail." Salinas added, "Then with a giggle a new chant was born: 'Your gloves don't match your shoes/You'll see it on the news.' "

Salinas reported that a rumor was making the rounds among the activists that Vice President George Bush had made some kind of offensive comment earlier that afternoon: "It was reported that he, too, had been booed while proclaiming his support for mandatory blood tests and that his response—clearly audible—was, 'There must be a gay group in here.' "

Salinas also reported that two of the drivers of the buses that ferried the protesters around D.C. "were allegedly approached by officials from the United States Health Service who, according to two of the drivers, apprised them of the 'danger' of their cargo. The drivers, who asked to remain anonymous, told the *Native* that they were informed that they were in danger of contagion by casual contact with anyone with AIDS, and that 'we should fumigate the buses when we get back to New York.' "

Salinas reported, in the same issue, that the Louisiana House of Representatives had "passed from committee a bill that would allow quarantining of persons who tested positive to HIV. . . . The bill, HB 1041, empowers the state's Department of Health and Human Resources (HHR) to obtain 'a civil arrest warrant' to indefinitely detain any person considered to be an 'imminent menace' to public health."

In his column, in the June 22 issue, Ed Sikov, our media reporter, critiqued disturbing pieces that had been written by two of America's leading public intellectuals, Norman Podhoretz and Nat Hentoff. On October 22, in the *New York Post*, Podhoretz had issued his own epidemiological challenge in a piece titled "AIDS Is Not a Risk For All." He wrote, "Is AIDS a danger to heterosexuals? In all probability the answer is no. Yet almost everything we hear—including a good deal of what is being said at the International Conference on AIDS in Washington this week—seems concentrated to create the impression that heterosexuals will soon be as much at risk as homosexuals already are." About the Podhoretz piece, Sikov wrote, "At great pains to prove that the world's public health experts are mere puppets, Podhoretz claims that most, if not all members of the often-cited 4% group of heterosexual AIDS cases bent on duping their doctors." Podhoretz would not be the only person to declare heterosexual AIDS a myth. In some ways it was a logical response to the politically crafted epidemiology the CDC was using to name and count cases of AIDS while turning a blind eye on the entire mostly-heterosexual chronic fatigue syndrome side of the AIDS equation. Podhoretz had the skeptical eye of an inquisitor when it came to the truthfulness of so-called heterosexual AIDS patients. He insisted, "Denials by AIDS patients of homosexual encounters cannot be taken at face value." It was a little like the CDC's logic which declared that if one had AIDS and one was HIV-negative, in reality, one was really HIV-positive by definition. Podhoretz was promoting one of the most toxic opposite world memes of the epidemic, that the gay community was actively engaged in a political conspiracy to promote politically correct epidemiology that *falsely* presented the epidemic as an equal opportunity plague. Podhoretz railed, "If heterosexual, white, middle-class Americans no longer regard AIDS as an imminent threat to them, the growing effort to contain it may falter."

In the same column, Sikov pointed out that with liberal friends like Nat Hentoff of the *Village Voice*, the gay community needed no enemies. In *The Washington Post*, on May 30, according to Sikov, "The former civil libertarian called for mandatory [HIV] testing." Sikov wrote, "Though his position flies in the face of what almost every public health expert tells us, Hentoff rages against those who fight compulsory testing and contact tracing. . . . Throughout the piece, Hentoff sets up a troubling dialectic between those who should be tested, their rights being sufficiently expendable, and the rest of the country, whose rights are more important. Opposition to mandatory testing [according to Hentoff] "results in violating the civil liberties of the unknowing victims of those who are victims of AIDS. These may well be termed violations caused by withholding crucial information from them.' This position stands solely on the idea that there can be innocent 'victims' of AIDS who acquired the disease in a funda-mentally different manner than those who are somehow more responsible for their fate."

Hentoff attacked the ACLU's position of supporting voluntary testing with strict confidentiality. Sikov argued, "Like many other anti-gay bigots who have jumped on the testing bandwagon, Hentoff labors under the delusion that it's possible to deny other people their civil rights while maintaining his own. For Hentoff, 'mandatory testing' does not mean that he would be subject to governmental intervention in his most private life; that's only for other people. His position will likely change when insurance companies and their friends in Congress, using compulsory 'AIDS testing' as a precedent, begin to agitate for mandatory testing for genetic predispositions to cancer, cystic fibrosis, and other illnesses. By then, however, it will be too late to quibble about who deserves civil rights."

In the July 6 issue of *New York Native,* we introduced the scientist Peter Duesberg to the world, in the form of a long interview by John Lauritsen. Lauritsen wrote, "The hypothesis that Human Immuno-deficiency Virus (HIV) the so-called 'AIDS virus' is the cause of AIDS may have been dealt a death blow by an article that appeared in the 1 March 1987 issue of *Cancer Research*: 'Retroviruses as Carcinogens and Pathogens: Expectations by Peter H. Duesberg.' The article broadly reviews the putative role of retroviruses (such as HTLV-I) in causing leukemia or other forms of cancer, as well as the role of HIV in causing AIDS. Duesberg concludes that it is far from proven that retroviruses play any role whatever in causing cancer, and that the claim that HIV causes AIDS is equally unfounded."

Lauritsen quoted Duesberg's judgment about HIV and AIDS from the *Cancer Research* article: "It seems likely that AIDS virus is just the most common occupational viral infections of AIDS patients and those at risk for AIDS rather than the cause of AIDS. The disease would then be caused by an as yet unidentified agent which may not even be a virus."

In the July 27 issue of *New York Native,* I wrote an article that challenged all of the epidemiological premises upon which conservative and liberal homophobes and heterosexists were basing their political attacks on gays. Titled "The Real Epidemic," I asked "Is AIDS actually an acute form of Chronic Epstein-Barr virus (CEBV) [another predecessor term for chronic fatigue syndrome]? That is bound to be the most urgent question to be settled by scientists in the months ahead. But other questions arise. Do CEBV and AIDS have the same cause, but different outcomes? Does every person who has AIDS have CEBV? And is the cause of CEBV Dr. Gallo's virus HBLV [eventually called HHV-6]?"

I reported, "In the May 30 issue of *Hospital Practice* magazine, Dr. Anthony L. Kamaroff, Director of the Division of General Medicine and Primary Care at Brigham and Women's Hospital, Harvard Medical School, gave one of the most complete descriptions of the syndrome called CEBV to date. Komaroff chooses to call the disorder Chronic Viral Fatigue Syndrome (CVFS). [Kamoroff's] report summarizes research performed on more than three hundred patients from various parts of the country who have chronic mononucleosis. . . . Komaroff concludes that CVFS [CEBV] is a real organic disease because of 'recurrent pharyngitis and other symptoms of upper respiratory infection, recurrent cervical adenopathy, and low grade fevers 99.4 to 100.4).' There are also striking neurological symptoms that occur in the first weeks of the illness. The symptoms improve but do not disappear. According to Komaroff, the patients generally describe the onset of symptoms in the same way. They were fine until one day 'they developed what seemed to be a simple "cold" or "flu" with sore throat, cervical adenopathy, myalgia (sometimes), gastrointestinal symptoms, fever and profound fatigue. But unlike any previous cold or flu, the illness never went away.' "

Regarding his notions about the cause and contagiousness of the syndrome, I reported, "Komaroff concludes that 'common exposure to some external agent, infectious or environmental, seems to be the unavoidable conclusion' because his research team found 'clusters of cases of affected persons who lived with one another and developed the illness at the same time.' " I also reported, "Komaroff admits that until the agent or agents which cause the disease are identified, diagnosis may be difficult." (One of the great understatements of all time.) I then stated what I thought was painfully obvious: "Because the cause of AIDS has not yet been established, the search for the cause of CVFS (CEBV) may also offer clues as to what causes AIDS because AIDS is so closely related to the syndrome. Two graphs which accompany Komaroff's article list the symptoms and clinical findings of people with CVFS (CEBV). People with AIDS show a number of these manifestations."

I also noted, "One scientist I talked to said that AIDS-related complex (ARC) is very much like [the syndrome Komaroff described]. Another referred to the syndrome as 'closet AIDS.' " I also pointed out, "As close readers of this newspaper would expect this writer to note, the question of the cause of CVFS (CEBV) may lead back to the virus which has been suggested as the cause of AIDS by some scientists: African swine fever virus. In pigs ASFV can cause acute disease (AIDS?) or chronic disease (CVFS/CEBV?)."

Had CEBV (chronic fatigue syndrome) been recognized as "closet AIDS" and been nudged out of its disingenuous closet, the pseudoscientific witch-hunt that intellectuals like Podhoretz and Hentoff were on might have been stopped in its tracks.

In that same issue of the paper, we reported again on the antics of New York City Councilman Joseph Lisa who was on that same bandwagon. Lisa had been considered for the leadership of the Council's Health Committee, but his name was withdrawn after he gave an interview to Joe Nicholson of the *New York Post* in which he reportedly said, "There are going to be instances of people who are out of control" that he thought should be quarantined. The *Post* had printed the story with a front page banner saying "AIDS Quarantine Urged." Another memorable moment in the abyss.

In that same issue of *New York Native*, we ran an interview with Gore Vidal by Terry Miller in which Vidal weighed in on AIDS and the state of the country: "You've got to remember, the aim of the government is to achieve total control over its citizens. Any government of any sort. It's instinctual. Drugs as an issue, was a godsend, so now they can have blood tests, and if you're in the government you have lie detector tests too. Have you been taking drugs? Now it's: Do you have AIDS? The idea is to create prohibitions and make *sure* that people break them. The government doesn't give a damn whether you take drugs, or go to bed with one another, or for that matter, whether you have AIDS or not. *They like the idea of control.* They want to have enough prohibitions so that they can, if they wish, put you in jail and *shut you up*. This is the hand our government plays, and not just with sex, but with everything."

In the August 10 issue, Mike Salinas reported on President Reagan's "National Advisory Panel to Address the Issues of the AIDS Epidemic." Salinas noted that many medical experts were stunned "by his appointments of men and women with little or no experience or prior experience with AIDS on any level." One AIDS activist called the commission a "death squad" and "the Inquisition." Salinas reported that the panel included a chairman "who had absolutely no AIDS experience, an Illinois legislator who had called for mandatory AIDS testing, a retired chief of naval operations who had called for mandatory testing and the president of a major corporation who was very active in right wing politics. One of the medical professionals on the panel was a regular guest host of televangelist Pat Robertson's program, *The 700 Club*." The wackiest appointee was probably "a sex therapist who favors abstinence as the best possible solution to the spread of AIDS." And, according to Salinas, "the panel's only ethnic minority member" was "the Health Commissioner for the state of Indiana who has used that position to call for the isolation of [HIV] seropositive individuals." The fact that there was also one openly gay appointee didn't make up for the disturbing fact that the panel also included John Cardinal O'Connor, Roman Catholic Archbishop of New York. Salinas noted that although O'Connor had personally volunteered to empty the bedpans of AIDS patients at St. Clare's Hospital in Manhattan, "He was also active in the fight to defeat Intro 2, the so-called 'gay rights bill' in New York City."

In the September 28 issue of the *Native*, we printed some of the testimony presented at the illustrious panel's first public meeting in Washington, D.C. While all of the testimony from AIDS activists was impassioned and perhaps well-meaning, like most of the thought-free activism of the epidemic, it was blind to the heterosexism that was the concrete foundation of the epidemic's epidemiology and the toxic public health agenda that it engendered.

Amy Ashworth, a well-known figure in Parents and Friends of Lesbians and Gays, told the committee, "On the Weekend of July 4, 1981, I first found out about AIDS. The *New York Times* had just a few lines mentioning a new disease that mostly attacked the gay community. I called my oldest son and told him my fears. I remember telling him that AIDS would become the worst plague, since prejudice against gays would prevent decisive action. Now I feel I have been living in two worlds: the terrible world of AIDS and the other, complacent world of those who ignore it. My fears were justified." (Ashworth's fear would be even more justified in the following years. Her only two sons, both gay, would die of AIDS.)

Bill Bahlman, a member of ACT UP and Lavender Hill Mob told the commission, "The use of placebo control trials in testing treatments for a life-threatening disease such as AIDS is highly immoral. Not only is it immoral, but persons with AIDS will not cooperate with placebo studies." (While this was driven by humanitarian intentions, it was a major threat to doing biomedical science that could be considered objective and trustworthy.

Scientifically speaking, it was sheer madness.) The good news was that he also criticized the government's obsession with AZT at the expense of other promising treatments for AIDS.

Martin Robinson, a member of ACT UP, also attacked the government for letting other drugs wait in line "behind a fleet of AZT studies." He called AZT the "dubious flagship of the NIH and the FDA." He insisted, "Seven years into the epidemic, scientific efforts that would lead to curative medicines are almost at ground zero." Ironically, given the subsequent legacy of the AIDS activists and the HIV establishment, he asked, "Who's to blame for this folly? Who has been complicitous? Are we suicidal? Are we genocidal? Medicine is the ethical response to AIDS, not opinion. There's no time. There's no time here for agendas—private agendas, using AIDS as a weapon." (Unfortunately. there was also no time for serious critical thinking on the part of either the establishment or the activists. And the AIDS activists had their own agenda.)

Henry Yeager, also a member of ACT UP and the Lavender Hill Mob, attacked mandatory HIV testing, arguing, "Since there is no cure for AIDS, no treatment, what does the government envision for people who test positive for HIV antibody? Incarceration? Warehousing? Quarantine? Attorney General Meese states publicly that HIV infection should be a factor in parole eligibility for incarcerated persons. In effect he is saying that people exposed to HIV belong in jail. At all government levels, there are proposals to legalize discrimination against [people with AIDS], people who test antibody positive, and even people perceived to be at risk for AIDS." While one can't find fault with sentiments like Yeager's, the baggage of epidemiological presumptions that usually came with such seemingly noble concerns were fated to sink the gay community into a hopeless quagmire of scientific mistakes and deceit. Like all AIDS activists, Yeager was a promoter of "education": "Only the radical modification of individual behavior will affect the trajectory of the AIDS epidemic. Such modification will only come, not from mandatory screening, but from a public commitment to the kind of sexual education that will entail an unprecedented willingness to suspend moralism in the name of life." This could be called a major gay "Stepin Fechit" moment (there were many) that most of the AIDS activists who spoke in public eventually performed, totally unaware that education which was based on the CDC's ersatz science. AIDS activism was essentially a great big gay minstrel show.

Larry Kramer, who billed himself as the co-founder of GMHC and the founder of ACT UP, also testified. He told the committee, "The field of AIDS research is a huge mess. It's strangled in bureaucratic red tape, inefficiency, and a lack of cooperation between people, agencies, and countries." Interestingly, Kramer told the commission that Dr. Anthony Fauci was being described "by many experts as 'in way over his head,' " and "the best scientists and researchers seem to be too scared to come anywhere near AIDS at all. Thus we're at the mercy of Drs. [Samuel] Broder and [Robert] Gallo of NIH, who use their positions of power to intimidate. Indeed, Gallo is known at NIH as 'the Godfather.' "

Once again, one thing AIDS Activist Numero Uno did not protest was the basic epidemiology and science that was employed in the construction of the HIV/AIDS paradigm. All the AIDS activists maintained an attitude of unquestioning, servile trust of the government's basic paradigm. Even in their angriest and most defiant moments their heads were bowed to the CDC's "homodemiology." Had the activists dared to accuse the government of not admitting that the emerging cases of CEBV or chronic fatigue syndrome were also part of the AIDS epidemic, it all would have turned out so differently. The gay and black communities might not have had to live with the yellow stars and scarlet letters of an HIV diagnosis.

In the same issue of *New York Native*, Charles Linebarger reported, "Northwest Orient Airlines refused to sell a ticket to the nation's capital to Leonard Matlovich, a Vietnam war hero and person with AIDS (PWA) who wishes to attend the October March on Washington for Lesbian and Gay Rights. Representatives of the local news media watched as ticket clerks and supervisors for the airlines explained to Matlovich that it is the airline's policy not to fly people who are believed to be infected with HIV, the so-called 'AIDS Virus.' "

In the October 19 issue, we ran one of the first hard-hitting exposés of the questionable AIDS treatment, AZT, by John Lauritsen. He analyzed a double-blind study of AZT that was published in the July 23, 1987, *New England Journal of Medicine*. Lauritsen wrote, "The description of methodology is incomplete and dishonest. Not a single table is acceptable according to statistical standards. Indeed not a single table makes sense."

The thing that upset Lauritsen the most was that the highly toxic drug was being given for "symptomatic HIV infection" when HIV hadn't even been proven to be the cause of AIDS. At the time Lauritsen was overly optimistic that the tide was turning against the HIV theory. He wrote, "The HIV edifice appears to have collapsed and the 'AIDS virus' crowd have resorted to stonewalling." Unfortunately that collapsing edifice stood for at least another quarter of a century.

The AZT study, as described by Lauritsen, sounded like a total unscientific mess: "The AZT trial was characterized throughout by sloppiness and lack of control. Recording forms were poorly designed, leading to confusion when doctors were asked to make judgments." Lauritsen argued that the seemingly impressive mortality data of the study did not stand up to scrutiny, pointing to "the inadequate descriptions of causes of death, the lack of verification of death causes, the lack of autopsies, and the refusal to release medical records." He concluded, "There is no doubt that AZT is a highly toxic drug, that it will be harmful to patients, many of whom are already severely debilitated. On the other hand, there is no scientifically credible evidence that AZT has any benefits whatsoever. The 'double blind, placebo-controlled' trial of AZT is unworthy of credence. . . . I submit that it is malpractice for physicians to prescribe AZT, a poison which can only harm the patient. I submit that it was unethical for AZT to be approved on the basis of research which was, to put it as generously as possible, invalid."

In the November 2 issue, we ran a *Bay Area Reporter* story by Jay Newquist who reported from California, "An AIDS scare campaign is being considered by state and national Republicans as a strategy to unseat Democrats who are sympathetic to the health crisis. A San Francisco political consulting firm under contract to the Republican Party has proposed a plan to 'incite public groundswell,' against Democratic candidates who are 'soft' on AIDS issues."

In the November 16 issue, I reported on a rather extraordinary event in the history of *New York Native*: "On November 2, I received a telephone called from Jim Warner, the Senior Policy Analyst in the Office of Policy Development in the White House. He had seen my name in an article in the September issue of the *Atlantic Monthly*. Warner knew that the *Native* has published a number of articles suggesting that HIV may not be the cause of AIDS, and he expressed concern that HIV may not adequately explain the epidemic. I asked

Warner about the President's position on the epidemic, and he told me that the President wants 'the best people to do the best thing,' but that the President doesn't feel that is being accomplished. Warner also told me that the White House could be seen as being divided into two groups on the issue of AIDS. One group, which he said is in the minority, wants to adopt an 'Auschwitz model' by quarantining all those infected with 'the virus.' 'The other group,' he said 'is incompetent.' Several times during our conversation, Warner stressed that there are many incompetent scientists working for the government. He said he was not impressed that a majority of scientists believe that HIV is the cause of AIDS, because throughout history majorities have been wrong. He is very concerned about the haphazard collection of data on HIV, and noted that between a million and a million-and-a-half Americans are 'infected.' If the epidemic is indeed spreading, Warner wonders why the CDC's estimates don't reflect it. Warner also asked me whether Dr. Robert Gallo (the man credited by some with the discovery of HIV, and by others with having stolen it from researchers at the Pasteur Institute in Paris) had ever stated that HIV is the cause of AIDS. I told him that Gallo had on numerous occasions. Warner expressed a desire to establish the real cause of AIDS so that the government resources could be spent on treating those infected. . . . Warner wanted to know how he could get in touch with Peter Duesberg, the retrovirologist who believes that Gallo is wrong about HIV's connection to AIDS. I gave him Duesberg's telephone number."

In the same issue, we published an article by Phil Zwickler about a fundraising letter that was being mailed to Manhattan businesses by a group called The Coalition for Public Health which was sponsored by The American Policy Institute. The letter was another example of the politically dystopian world that AIDS had become. The very nasty and hypocritical political letter accused the gay community of playing politics with the epidemic. The letter, according to Zwickler's report, called "on all New Yorkers to get involved in stopping the spread of AIDS." And it promoted "mandatory AIDS testing." The word "mandatory" had become a menacing rhetorical baseball bat through-out the epidemic.

In the December 7 issue of *New York Native,* we published the text of a speech that was given by Larry Kramer at the Sixth Annual Human Rights Campaign Fund Dinner at the Waldorf Astoria Hotel in

Manhattan. Kramer said, "In reading over my collected diatribes of the past years, I realized I am still unable to resolve this fundamental problem: how to inspire you without punishing you." (Kramer was from the bizarre school of speakers who announce what effect they are going to have on you. ACT UP was cut from the same presumptuous cloth in that the organization often announced what impact their actions were having. It was never left to observers or historians. It really was just another way of telling the gay community what they were supposed to be thinking.) Kramer noted in his talk, "We have managed to turn mourning into some kind of art form," making one wonder just how authentic that kind of mourning really was.

Kramer once again pontificated on a litany of the gay community's failures: "We are woefully unprepared;" "We still have no leaders with national recognition;" "We still have not learned how to broker our power;" "We still have no national publication that is worthy of respect;" "We still have no national organizations that are strong."

One of Kramer's questionable themes was always the lack of cooperation between gay and AIDS groups and the constant pedestrian demand that they "consolidate." In retrospect, during the epidemic, there was *too much* cooperation between gay groups, which turned them into one big unthinking gay blob.

Ironically, considering the salient theme of this book, Kramer said, "In my writing, I make a lot of comparisons between gays now and the Jewish community before the war. The Jews thought of themselves as good Germans first and good Jews second. When the horror started, they couldn't believe what their fellow Germans were doing to them." The irony here is of course that at least the Jews could eventually see what was actually transpiring around them, but the epidemiologically clueless Kramer and his ilk were totally blind to what was really happening to the gay community—with their help. Kramer argued, "The battle is first and foremost for a cure." That sounds good, but that battle was secondary to a far more important one Kramer didn't even know he should have been fighting, a battle for the whole truth about the real epidemic that was concealed by heterosexist epidemiology that created the demonic public health paradigm.

Kramer does deserve some credit for calling Anthony Fauci "Public Enemy Number One" in the speech. He accused Fauci of setting up treatment centers that did not work and of squandering millions of dollars on studies of AZT. Kramer was constantly screaming murder and genocide without himself really understanding what the primary source of the murder and the genocide actually was. In the speech he also said, "Oh, my people, why don't you hear me when I use the word 'murdered?' Why don't you believe me when I tell you that Dr. Fauci and his boss, Dr. Wyngaarden, and our president, Ronald Reagan, and our Mayor Edward I. Koch—all megalomaniacs playing god—are murdering us?" The only thing one can say about this list is that it is a judgment-free collection of apples and oranges. In many ways Ed Koch, who Kramer was oddly obsessed with and often accused of being a closet homosexual, was considered at that time to be a reliable friend of the gay community. As far as Kramer's charge of "megalomaniacs" goes, it was coming from the inside of a glass house.

In the same issue of the *Native*, we published an article by Ed Koch which was sent to us by his office in response to Kramer's speech. In it Koch attacked anti-gay members of Congress for trying to pass an amendment to an AIDS bill that would declare, "None of the federal money that is appropriated to the Centers for Disease Control in Atlanta can be used directly or indirectly for propagating or expanding directly or indirectly the homosexual lifestyle." The amendment was an indirect attack on Gay Men's Health Crisis which, ironically, through its education efforts was itself propagating the government's scapegoating epidemiology and AIDS paradigm. The right-wing Congressmen should have been cheering the propaganda efforts of GMHC.

In the December 28 issue, we published an update on AZT by John Lauritsen. He reported that despite the growing doubts about the safety and efficacy of AZT, "Doctors in New York have become even more aggressive in persuading and even bullying their patients into taking AZT. I have twice had the gut-wrenching experience of talking to young men who are healthy, although they have tested positive for antibodies to HIV and have low T-cell ratios, trying to dissuade them from going on AZT. Both times I failed. They agreed with everything I said, but the bottom line was that they trusted their doctors."

Lauritsen also reported that he was "now investigating a report of a young man, admitted to a New York hospital with his first case of Pneumocystis carinii pneumonia, was immediately put on AZT, despite his strong objections. If this report is true, then fundamental questions of medical ethics are involved. Do doctors have the right to force a patient against his will to take a highly toxic drug whose benefits are entirely speculative?"

1988: The Public Relations of the Epidemic

The new year brought with it the hope that a meeting scheduled by James Warner for a debate about whether HIV was a huge scientific mistake would actually take place in the White House. Warner had invited both Peter Duesberg and Robert Gallo to the meeting. But, on January 8, Joe Nicholson reported in the *New York Post* that the meeting had been canceled.

Ironically, a man who was no friend of the gay community, Gary Bauer, President Reagan's top domestic adviser, was a sponsor of the meeting and was concerned that HIV might not be the cause of AIDS. Nicholson reported that Bauer told him, "I've sort of bristled at the finality with which some have made statements about AIDS and how it is transmitted. When findings run counter to accepted wisdom, there is a tendency to muzzle or ignore rather than have an open debate."

Harvey Bialy, who was a research editor at *Bio/Technology* magazine and was a supporter of Peter Duesberg's criticism of HIV, had been called by the White House to help organize the meeting. Bialy had suggested that the White House invite Gallo and Fauci to the debate. In his book, *Oncogenes, Aneuploidy, and AIDS: A Scientific Life and Times of Peter H. Duesberg*, Bialy wrote, "The day of our 1987 Christmas office party, I spoke with Jim Warner for the last time when he called to tell me that sadly the meeting was off. He had been advised that Anthony Fauci, far from reacting as I anticipated, threw a 'snit fit' when he was invited, and demanded to know why the White House was interfering in scientific matters that belonged to NIH and the Office of Scientific and Technology Assessment. . . . I always thought that the short-circuiting of the scientific meeting was a watershed moment in the battle over the etiology of AIDS." In retrospect, had it happened, it might have altered the course of AIDS/CFS history. But for AIDS dissidence, bad luck seemed to rule the day.

In one of the more bizarre chapters in the *Native*'s history, Ann Fettner, who had done such an astounding job of exposing the deceitful nature of the CDC's science (for which I am eternally grateful), suddenly got HIV religion and in a shocking betrayal of everything I thought she stood for, she wrote a piece attacking Duesberg, in the February 2 issue of the *Village Voice*. In my editorial response, I wrote, "On the subject of the epidemic, the *Voice* gets stranger and stranger. Those of us who used to love the *Voice* because it spoke truth to power are in a state of shock that the paper has been turned . . . into a house organ for the government's line of baloney on the epidemic. As far as Fettner is concerned, I have to take the blame for having created a monster. But I do think that most of what she wrote for the *Native* had—and still has—merit. The idea of Fettner treating Duesberg as if he were some kind of crackpot is absurd. Everybody in the field of retrovirology knows that he is a serious scientist, and that his ideas are anything but frivolous. The same cannot be said about Fettner's [new] 'scientific' ideas." In her *Voice* piece, Fettner quoted the ever-petulant Fauci as saying that major AIDS researchers would not take Duesberg seriously because "they're much too busy, they've got too much to do to do that."

Fettner was on a personal mission that was clearly driven by a certain amount of spite towards me for not being able to afford to keep her writing for the *Native*. She now mocked the whole idea of African swine fever being the cause of AIDS, framing it as just a grand conspiracy theory. (She wouldn't be the first to concoct that tactic to try and permanently stigmatize the idea.) According to her, "HIV is fabulous enough to provide all the answers needed to explain the equally fabulous disease it kicks off." Such cogent thinking is why the epidemic turned out to be such a "fabulous" time for all involved. It's tragic to think that if the *Native* had not been hanging by a financial thread and I had enough money to pay her to write for the *Native* she might never have ended up on the HIV bandwagon, attacking virtually the only publication (other than *Spin*, a monthly magazine which published Celia Farber's excellent investigative journalism) that dared to do any critical reporting on the epidemic.

In the February 29 issue, John Lauritsen penned a critical piece about the way the *Voice* and Fettner handled the Duesberg story, starting with the intentionally nasty way the paper photographed Duesberg. He wrote, "The *Voice* sent a team of photographers to shoot Duesberg in Berkeley. They treated him like royalty, shot him in many different poses and left. After an hour, they returned and took still more shots. After all that, the photograph published in the *Voice* shows Duesberg leaning forward, his hand stretching toward the camera, his eyes almost closed, his expression tense. The camera angle is grotesquely lopsided. The lighting is harsh, from the side and below—

the kind of lighting known as 'monster lighting,' because of its use in horror movies. The photo makes Duesberg look sinister and demented—like a 'mad scientist' from a cheaply made science-fiction/horror movie. In fact Duesberg is a very photogenic man. I have photographed him on two occasions and found it almost effortless to obtain excellent portraits. . . . All photographs need not be flattering, but they should at least be truthful. The *Village Voice* published a photograph that does not look anything like Duesberg: a cheap propaganda trick."

Lauritsen reported that when Fettner "interviewed Duesberg, she flattered him in every way, agreed with him again and again, and indicated that she was simply thrilled to be talking to such an important scientist. . . . Out of a long interview she conducted, Fettner quotes only a few sentences of Duesberg's, and these are hopelessly mangled and out of context. . . . From Fettner's article, no one would know what Duesberg's ideas are, or where to find them. Fettner doesn't want the reader to know. . . . After spewing out quite a bit of impertinent and distasteful gossip, Fettner suddenly shifts gears and goes into rather wild speculation on ways in which HIV might cause AIDS. . . . Fettner concludes her piece by accusing Duesberg of holding back the fight against AIDS. With so much new research being generated, and so much that needs to be done, she asks, why are we now forced to stop and deal with Duesberg's passé propositions? Fettner's accusation is despicable. All that is being asked of Gallo, Fauci, Haseltine, Essex and Montagnier, is that they fulfill their obligations as scientists and defend their hypothesis, in an appropriate publication, against Duesberg's critique."

In the March 21 issue, in an editorial, I brought up the matter of the possible relationship between HHV-6 and African swine fever: "As most readers of this newspaper know, I presume that the large DNA virus with which Robert Gallo is currently playing science is African swine fever virus. As data leaks out of his lab, it's clear that his virus is linking itself to both chronic fatigue syndrome and Acquired Immunodeficiency Syndrome. People like Howard Streicher, Gallo's charming Guy Friday, hem and haw about not having a good test for their swine virus, and have therefore come to no conclusions. But discussions with a source close to the heart of their research suggest a necessary cofactor for AIDS has been found. If that's true, Gallo's African swine fever virus could also become a nominee for the "cause" of AIDS. Perhaps African swine fever is the pathogen toward which we should be directing our vaccine and antiviral efforts. And shouldn't we be screening the blood supply for African swine fever virus if it is a cofactor of AIDS and a cause of chronic fatigue syndrome? Gallo's biggest problem with his [recently discovered] virus is that it destroys cells in the immune system more efficiently than his Human Immunodeficiency Virus (HIV). The pathogenic difference between the two viruses is so dramatic that one well-known scientist in New York is reported to have said that if Gallo's DNA virus had been discovered before his RNA virus, it would have been declared the cause of AIDS."

I also wrote, "One of the more amusing developments in swine fever research involves scientist Jane Teas and British researcher Robert G. Downing. Several years ago, Downing helped Teas test blood from AIDS patients for the presence of several strains of African swine fever virus. As we have reported in these pages, the tests [performed in England] were positive for a number of samples. Teas flew back to the U.S. expecting to write up the results with Downing and submit them to a medical journal. But over the ensuing weeks, Downing wouldn't acknowledge her phone calls, and their collaboration fell apart. But Downing suddenly resurfaced in the August 15, 1987, issue of *The Lancet*, where he reported on the isolation of a large, DNA virus from AIDS patients in Uganda. And what does he call it? A 'human herpesvirus.' [It was of course the virus that turned out to be HHV-6.] Based on a conversation I had last year with a senior member of the U.S Department of Agriculture, I've come to think that Gallo and Downing's basic game plan is to exploit the limited similarities between African swine fever virus and cytomegalovirus (CMV), another DNA virus for which ASFV has been mistaken, to keep the public from knowing the truth about AIDS and chronic fatigue syndrome. The last time I talked to Gallo, he was not too happy about Downing. I would be wary of him, too, since he's familiar with the Teas [ASFV] data and could expose the truth about Gallo's virus whenever he wants."

I also noted, "The emergence of a new cause or co-cause of AIDS will add to the credibility of retrovirologist Peter Duesberg's theory. Duesberg has challenged the orthodoxy that HIV is the cause of AIDS. . . . In a related matter, we must all try to educate ourselves about the plight of people affected by chronic fatigue syndrome. Their suffering is enormous. My discussions with students of the chronic fatigue syndrome epidemic suggest that its breadth dwarfs the AIDS epidemic considerably. And although it may not seem as acute, it may be creating a nation of chronically ill men and women. Chronic fatigue syndrome is still in the closet, partly due to the politics of HHV-6 and African swine fever virus, but it is expected to get a media boost from Congressional hearings in the months ahead. Chronic fatigue syndrome should be declared a priority health problem by the National Institutes of Health. Funding for chronic fatigue syndrome research is miniscule and the public knows little about the disease. . . . People with the illness exhibit a wide array of unusual symptoms and clinical problems. Cancer and circulatory problems can occur. Most ominous is the neurological damage that some researchers have encountered. People with the syndrome sometimes have trouble concentrating and make perceptual mistakes."

In the same issue of the *Native*, we ran an article by Phil Zwickler about the reaction to a book by Dr. William H. Masters, his partner Virginia Johnson, and Dr. Robert Kolodny. *Crisis: Heterosexual Behavior in the Age of AIDS*, which was published by Grove Press. The authors concluded, "Authorities are greatly underestimating the number of people infected with the AIDS virus in the population today." The writers had strayed off the AIDS reservation and dared to tell truths which came very close to outing the real epidemic behind the political veil of the HIV epidemic. Zwickler wrote, "While stating that AIDS is 'now running rampant in the heterosexual community,' they maintain that three million Americans, more than twice the number claimed by public health experts, are seropositive." The authors shocked the nation by asserting, "Infection with the AIDS virus does not require intimate sexual contact or sharing of intravenous needles; transmission can, and does, occur as a result of person-to-person contact in which blood or other body fluids from a person who is harboring the virus are splashed onto or rubbed against someone else."

Masters, Johnson, and Kolodny seem to have inadvertently glanced into *something closer to the real epidemic* and were more in touch with what was going on behind the jerry-built paradigm than even they realized. They paid a price for trying to tell it like it is. A series of reactions gathered by Zwickler did a stunning job of catching in real time the vicious political correctness that was forming around the government's paradigm. It also showed how an unholy alliance between AIDS activists, quasi-governmental AIDS organizations and the gay community was forming. Masters, Johnson, and Kolodny had called for something draconian which helped cement an unholy alliance of opposition. According to Zwickler, "The authors call for mandatory HIV antibody testing for couples seeking a marriage license, pregnant women, convicted prostitutes, and all hospital in-patients between the ages of 15 and 60, as a way of stopping the epidemic."

Dr. Stephen Joseph, the New York City Commissioner of Health, told Zwickler that the authors raised "all the old 'bugaboos' about transmission." Interestingly, Joseph inadvertently caught the constantly shifting landscape of information about the epidemic when he said, "The book is damaging in that it takes us off on a swing. In the media, nine months ago, a heterosexual explosion of AIDS was cited. Three months ago *Cosmopolitan* said heterosexuals were not at risk. Now, Masters and Johnson write this book. It does confuse people. Heterosexual transmission is a real problem, but rampant spread, an image of diffuse spread—that's not happening." That was of course very true if you didn't factor chronic fatigue syndrome into the paradigm of AIDS. If the public was confused, it is because of the unsteadiness and lack of consistency at the very heart of the public relations image of the epidemic that the CDC was promoting. Masters, Johnson, and Kolodny were hopelessly trying to make sense out of a paradigm that was half self-deception and half noble epidemiological lie meant to keep everybody pacified.

Mathilde Krim, the founding chair of the American Foundation for AIDS Research, told Zwickler, "I believe it is an insult for Dr. Virginia Johnson to suggest that the time-tested methods of medical investigation have resulted in 'benevolent scientific deceptiveness' concerning AIDS, its modes of transmission and its rate of transmission." Peter Drotman, an epidemiologist with the CDC's AIDS Program told Zwickler, "The book is not helpful. It is not a scientific contribution to our understanding of AIDS. It stresses some far-fetched scenarios that seem designed to provoke anxiety rather than to make useful suggestions. . . . AIDS is pretty clearly not running rampant among heterosexuals." He was right of course because the form of acquired immunodeficiency that was running rampant in the heterosexual population was simply renamed chronic fatigue syndrome. Epidemiological rebranding was an instant cure for AIDS in the heterosexual population.

Unfortunately, the gay people Zwickler interviewed performed like a perky backup chorus to the AIDS establishment. Christopher Babick, Acting Director of People With AIDS Coalition, said, "I think their book is a reckless piece of literature. AIDS continues to affect mostly the communities it always has—namely, gay men, IV-drug users and their sexual partners." Maria Maggenti of the Women's Committee, AIDS Coalition to Unleash Power went even further, telling the *Native*, "I'm pretty horrified by the whole thing. Major actions should be taken against the book because it is only fueling the misinformation out there." (The gay community developed a very unfortunate and self-destructive taste for "major action" censorship during the epidemic.) Lori Behrman, the spokesperson for Gay Men's Health Crisis said, "Masters and Johnson have squandered their credibility to exploit a grave public health issue. Every AIDS researcher in the country will tell you that HIV cannot be transmitted casually. Their conclusion that mandatory testing is the answer overlooks the less expensive, more effective tool, which is education. The gay community has proved that safer sex and not testing can provide protection." In truth, the least expensive and most effective tool was actually the CDC's political epidemiology, which used public relations and a biased anti-gay paradigm to keep the disease from *appearing* to spread in the general population. This was just another example of the gay community having to do its abject "education is protection" minstrel show in the face of the draconian, spiteful call for mandatory testing. Every time the word "mandatory" was used it had more than a nasty little soupçon of "Get the gays" to it. The gay community, in such a dire situation, had to make a pact with the AIDS establishment to accept all the elements of its very political epidemiology—or else! Had the gay community called it out for the biased "homodemiology" that it was, everything would have been different.

Masters, Johnson, and Kolodny were threatening to expose what Daniel Goleman (after Ibsen) refered to as a "vital lie" which, Goleman describes as "a family myth that stands in place of a less comfortable truth." In this case it was a "vital lie" about the AIDS epidemic that prevented social anxiety. In Zwickler's survey of the AIDS and gay elite, one could see the social construction of a comforting false reality, a psychological phenomenon explored at length in Goleman's book, *Vital Lies, Simple Truths*. This moment in the epidemic captures Goleman's central thesis: "We are piloted in part by an ingenious capacity to deceive ourselves, whereby we sink into obliviousness rather than face threatening facts. This tendency to self-deception and mutual pretense pervades the structure of psychological life."

You could say that a kind of conspiracy of self-deception had begun on a massive scale in America and Masters, Johnson, and Kolodny (like the *Native*) were playing the role of unwelcome truth-tellers who needed to be neutralized by a kind of thuggish mockery. This moment was yet more evidence that, during the epidemic, there was never any such thing as what Goleman refers to as "acceptable dissent."

In the March 28 issue, we published John Lauritsen's most hard-hitting attack on AZT titled "AZT Iatrogenic Genocide." Lauritsen complained that five months after his first exposé of AZT, "the same old lies continue to appear in the mainstream press. It is still claimed that AZT 'extends life.' AZT not only continues to be marketed, but is being promoted more heavily than ever. In New York City, nearly all doctors with an AIDS practice are prescribing AZT, some of them indiscriminately. According to an article by Gina Kolata, in the *New York Times* (December 21, 1987), some doctors " 'have no set guidelines but let the patients decide if they want the drug.' " One wonders what the government would have done if the gay community had decided en masse *not* to take the drug. What if there had been an AZT version of the Boston Tea Party?

The tragedy of the epidemic was captured in technicolor by Lauritsen: "Not all patients have taken AZT voluntarily. Some have been bullied into taking it by their doctors. In Trenton State Prison, prisoners are being forced to take AZT against their will. In St. Vincent's Hospital, a patient's request not to be given AZT was ignored. And in Chicago, a hospitalized AIDS patient was declared insane because of his refusal to take AZT; the doctors said his refusal meant he didn't want to live and he was forced to take AZT."

Lauritsen was shocked at the course of events and his critique of what was going on was devastating: "It isn't supposed to happen like this. In fiction or the movies, once the crime and the criminal have been exposed, the plot is almost over. The malefactors are apprehended and brought to justice. End of story. But in real life, when your opponent is a wealthy, powerful, and unscrupulous drug manufacturer, who is aided and abetted by the stupidity, venality, and authoritarianism of the medical profession, the struggle goes on and on. A reasoned analysis, backed up by plenty of evidence, is countered with a propaganda juggernaut (advertising campaign) that shows total contempt for reason and evidence. And it works. Most people forget about facts if they haven't heard them repeated within the past few weeks (or days)."

Lauritsen summed up the AZT situation at that point: "We know for sure that AZT is a highly toxic drug, so toxic that about half of all AIDS patients cannot tolerate it and have to be taken off the drug. AZT destroys bone marrow and causes anemia so severe as to necessitate frequent transfusions. We know that AZT is cytotoxic—it kills healthy cells. We know that AZT attacks DNA synthesis. . . . In San Francisco, where doctors are more critical of AZT, doctors admit to having seen horrible results from AZT: liver, kidney, and neurological damage as well as the inevitable anemia and trans-fusions."

Lauritsen also noted, "On February 19, 1988, Dr. Anthony Fauci of the National Institutes of Allergy and Infectious Diseases, who is in charge of federal AIDS funding, appeared on the television program *Good Morning, America*. (Prof. Peter Duesberg was also to have appeared on the program, in order to debate Fauci on whether HIV causes AIDS, but he was disinvited at the last moment, for reasons that have yet to be explained.) Fauci was asked why only one drug had been made available. He replied, 'The reason that only one drug has been made available—AZT—is because it's the only drug that has been shown in scientifically controlled trials to be safe and effective.' " Lauritsen noted, "This brief statement contains several falsehoods. (Since I don't know whether Fauci told these untruths deliberately or out of ignorance, I'll simply call them 'falsehoods,' as opposed to 'lies.') First . . . there have been no 'scientifically controlled trials' of AZT. Second, AZT is not 'safe.' It is a highly toxic drug (the FDA analyst who reviewed the toxicology data recommended that AZT should not be approved). Third, AZT is not known objectively to be 'effective' for anything, except perhaps causing anemia, destroying bone marrow, and blocking DNA synthesis."

Lauritsen came to a very dark conclusion: "It is difficult to avoid thinking that we gay men have been targeted for destruction. . . . At this point, we don't know the long term effects of AZT; no one has taken it for more than two years. However, death within a few years would appear to be the consequence of a drug that causes severe anemia, destroys bone marrow, and blocks DNA synthesis."

The unmitigated horror of the epidemic was also caught in Lauritsen's report that Dr. William Haseltine of the Dana Farber Institute in Boston told the Presidential Committee on AIDS on February 19 that AZT should be given to all members of 'high risk' groups." Lauritsen wrote, "His reasoning was as follows: 'HIV infection' is still confined to the present risk groups, gay men and IV-drug users. However, uninfected gay men face an annual risk of becoming infected, and this in turn represents a threat to the general population. Therefore, as a containment measure, HIV-antibody negative gay men should be given AZT in order to prevent their becoming 'infected.' " Lauritsen asserted, "Haseltine's analysis is based on the probably false premise that HIV is the cause of AIDS. It assumes that AZT kills or somehow inhibits HIV, whereas there is no evidence that it does. Everything about Haseltine's suggestion is wrong, unless one believes it is a good thing to kill off gay men and other members of 'risk groups.' "

Lauritsen then let out a clarion call for which he deserves a special place in history: "It's time for us to wake up. Healthy gay men are being targeted for genocide. Why do we let them do this to us? Where is our anger? We have become numb: From mourning, when we couldn't mourn. From held-in-rage and disgust at the lies, the greed, the malice, and the incompetence of those we ought to be able to depend on. From unrelenting fear, from confusion, from not knowing what to do. Our wills have become paralyzed."

He continued, "We must act to prevent our brothers from being poisoned. The time has come to express our anger. The time has come for us to be honest with our friends who have been gulled into taking AZT. We should tell them, tactfully but directly, that they are being poisoned, and that if necessary, they should change directions."

He closed his piece by declaring, "AZT doctors should be sued for engaging in false and misleading advertising. Public Health Service officials should be sued for unethical and illegal conduct. The time has come for lawsuits."

Earlier in 1988, I had hired a woman named Neenyah Ostrom as my assistant. She had been working at Biogen in Boston and, for a while, was the assistant to Walter Gilbert, a Nobel Prize Winner. She had originally pursued a career in medicine but decided during her pre-med courses that it wasn't for her. I was so impressed with her intelligence and editorial talents that soon after I hired her I asked her to begin covering chronic fatigue syndrome on a regular basis for *New York Native*. I also chose to do this as a way of sending a signal to the AIDS establishment that we were absolutely not going to back down on our concern that CFS and AIDS were totally intertwined. We made her work a regular feature and gave her column the title "Chronic Fatigue Report." The *New York Native* thorn in the AIDS establishment's side was about to become more painful.

Ostrom's first article was titled "Movement in Search of a Name." The piece began, "A new disease is ravaging our country. An increasing number of people are no longer able to work, to care for their families or themselves. They suffer from fevers, sore throats, swollen lymph glands, depression, headaches, neurological dysfunction, memory loss, cognitive disorders. Some develop brain lesions; some, B-cell lymphomas. Pervading all these symptoms is an overwhelming exhaustion that leaves patients unable to lift a toothbrush, stand long enough to shower, or even get out of bed. These frightened, exhausted people deplete their savings in search of medical care. In desperation, they go from one physician to another, most of whom are unable to diagnose their illness or—even more devastating—pronounce it to be psychosomatic."

Ostrom then asked a question that would be asked continuously for the next quarter of a century: "In this age of lasers and holography, when it has become routine to rearrange the DNA of living organisms, how is it possible that a debilitating new disease is falling through the cracks of scientific inquiry?"

Ostrom reported, "Chronic Epstein-Barr virus (CEBV) syndrome was the name given to the outbreak that brought the illness to national attention, a mini-epidemic near Lake Tahoe, Nevada, in 1985." She noted that the name was falling into disfavor because it was becoming clear that EBV was not the cause. She then cut to the chase and made a point that would be maintained by the newspaper until its demise in 1997: "But what has most impeded research has been the (recently reversed) refusal of the Federal Centers for Disease Control" to acknowledge the syndrome's existence. Ted Van Zelst, a philanthropist who had created an organization to fund research into the syndrome told her, "The CDC took the position very adamantly until mid-1986 that no such disease existed."

Ostrom wrote that at that point an organization for sufferers of the syndrome had "12,000 paid members and more than 200 local chapters across the U.S." A leader of the San Francisco chapter of that organization, Jan Montgomery, told Ostrom that the "illness does not stand alone, but is part of a group of immunosuppressive syndromes, including, but not limited to, AIDS and AIDS-related complex." (It was, as we shall see, a rare moment of unflinching honesty from a CFS patient and activist.)

At that time, according to Ostrom, "The two names the association is considering for the disease" were "Chronic Fatigue Immune Dysfunction Syndrome and Acquired Chronic Immune Dysfunction." The use of the word "fatigue" was already seen as a serious scientific and political mistake. Ostrom wrote, "The people I discussed it with at several local CEBV Association chapters were unanimous about eradicating 'fatigue' from the description, because of the trivializing effect. Overwhelming fatigue is a symptom, along with flu-like symptoms such as fever, swollen glands, sore throat, headaches, muscle aches and depression. These symptoms don't go away for months, sometimes years. In some cases, there is a progression to extreme mental and neurological deterioration, lesions in the brain, and a rare form of a fatal malignancy, B-lymphotropic cancer."

Ostrom also reported that the CDC's Dr. Gary Holmes had been dismissive of the disease in the *New York Times* and *Hippocrates Magazine* where he blamed the fuss on the media and physicians who got caught up in a kind of mania and started seeing and diagnosing the disease everywhere.

The scope of the epidemic was controversial then in 1988 and remained so for the next 25 years. Ostrom pointed out that in a *JAMA* article in May of 1987, Harvard scientist Anthony Kamaroff "reported major symptoms of chronic fatigue syndrome in 21% of 500 randomly selected hospital patients."

In mid-April, the *New York Times* and *The Washington Post* published stories raising questions about the scientific integrity of David Baltimore, a Nobel Prize winner and someone who was part of the nation's AIDS inner circle. I wrote in the *Native*, "A research paper published by Baltimore and others is not backed by research which they conducted, and Baltimore refused to retract the paper and has done everything he can to hurt the career of a scientist who discovered his phony conclusions. The pattern emulates the behavior of Harvard School of Publish Health researcher Myron Essex when scientists began to find that an antigen called F.O.C.M.A., which Essex 'discovered,' does not really exist. Soon their careers did not exist."

I took the opportunity to raise a larger issue: "The possibility that Baltimore is a con artist doesn't help the case of HIV, which he has been backing for some time. Fraud seems to be a way of life among scientists who are in charge of AIDS research in this country. One of the key questions Congress needs to ask is whether the domination of American AIDS research by scientific crooks such as Essex, Baltimore, and Robert Gallo, and incompetents such as Samuel Broder, Anthony Fauci, and Harold Jaffe, has discouraged scientists with brains and integrity from getting involved. Who would want to work in a scientific cesspool in which you get fired or lose grants because you tell the truth?"

I then laid out the case for HHV-6 being the new politically correct name for African swine fever virus: "As the papers about a virus called human herpesvirus-6 (HHV-6) slowly appear (and there is some speculation that the White House has ordered HHV-6 papers to emerge slowly), it looks like the cause of AIDS will turn out to be that virus (or a related DNA virus), and *not* HIV. The trail of epidemiology and lab research also leads to this conclusion: HHV-6 will turn out to be African swine fever virus. Jane Teas will turn out to have been correct when she hypothesized that African swine fever virus causes AIDS, and Gallo and Luc Montagnier will turn out to be wrong. (Teas has not publicly posited the theory that African swine fever virus is the cause of chronic fatigue syndrome, but the *Native* has.) Teas has found it difficult to find a job in science as a result of the promulgation of her ideas. If she turns out to be correct, she deserves every scientific award imaginable, and a major position at the scientific institution of her choice. It is worth pointing out that the person who noted the errors in Baltimore's research paper was a woman, too. Women who tell the truth don't fare well in American science."

I also let Mathilde Krim have it in the editorial: "In *Omni* magazine's November 1987 issue, Mathilde Krim said, 'In today's system of science, I think at the top there is less difference between men and women because those of both sexes who are different have already been eliminated. At the top all have learned to play the same game. And it's a bit of a con game.' My question to Krim is: Which con game are you and the American Foundation for AIDS Research playing this week? How difficult would it be for amfAR to admit that AIDS research has revolved around the wrong virus for five years, and that we have a lot of work to do with African swine fever virus? The best course of action at this point would be not to continue throwing good money after bad. Krim has an opportunity to lead our nation out of this huge scientific mistake. Americans can live with mistakes, but will face total catastrophe if the lies about African swine fever virus continue much longer."

I asserted, "Gallo's scam of trying to sell African swine fever virus as HHV-6 is yet another example of his crookedness. He doesn't want Teas to get credit for figuring out the cause of AIDS from both her epidemiology and the lab work she did with researchers John Beldekas and James Hebert. Gallo's lies are dangerous to himself, his staff, and the nation. A source close to Gallo's staff has told the *Native* that the wife of one of Gallo's associates is sick with the chronic disease (CFS) that may be caused by African swine fever virus. Is Gallo telling the poor woman that she's infected with HHV-6, when in reality she's suffering from a chronic infection with swine fever virus—which is absolutely *not* a herpesvirus. (Even Dr. Pearson of George Washington University told me that they're not certain [HHV-6 is] a herpesvirus.)"

Again the eternal optimist who thought change was right around the corner, I wrote, "There are at a least dozen scientists in America who have done extensive research on African swine fever virus. They should be summoned to the National Institutes of Health to help the nation figure out what to do about the virus Gallo tried to con the nation into believing was a herpesvirus."

In her "Chronic Fatigue Report" in the same issue, Neenyah Ostrom introduced the *Native* readers to Stephen E. Straus of the National Institute of Allergy and Infectious Diseases (NIAID), the man who would become public enemy number one to CFS patients and activists. Straus was in charge of what NIAID called its CFS research for the formative years of the CFS epidemic or cover-up, depending on your point of view. Ostrom reported, "Straus remains a vocal proponent of the psychoneurotic theory of CFS. In his [*JAMA*] March 1988 article he states, 'It is impossible to completely dispel the notion that the chronic fatigue syndrome represents a psychoneurotic condition. On the contrary, there are observations that support the hypothesis.' Straus cites an outbreak of 'mass hysteria' at the Royal Free Hospital in London in 1955. He also references the unpublished observations of Dr. Markus Kruesi at the National Institutes of Health that psychiatric evaluations of patients with CFS reveal that a 'very high proportion' have a history of depression, phobias or anxiety disorders. His article concludes: 'Ultimately, any hypothesis regarding the cause of the chronic fatigue syndrome must incorporate the psycho-pathology that accompanies and, in some cases, precedes it.' "

In the same report, Ostrom noted that early testing of CFS patients for HHV-6 was not producing any clear-cut results. (Testing would turn out to be a persistent political and scientific problem for the virus.)

She noted, "Because four of the six patients from whom HHV-6 initially was isolated had B cell cancers similar to those seen in CFS, a number of investigators suggested that HHV-6 might be the cause of CFS. Reports have appeared in the press that one of the Incline Village physicians, [Paul] Cheney, sent blood samples to Gallo's lab to be assayed for HHV-6." Cheney wasn't specific but told Ostrom the results were disappointing. Ostrom also reported, "In a March 1988 article in *Journal of Experimental Medicine*, Stephen Straus of NIAID quotes unpublished observations about HHV-6 from Gallo's laboratory. According to Straus, antibodies to HHV-6 are found in 10%-40% of 'normal American adults,' and in 6-80% of patients with AIDS, B cell lymphomas, and CFS. Despite the high prevalence, and 'relatively insensitive' serological methods, Straus concludes that HHV-6 remains an orphan virus in search of a disease.' "

"Relatively insensitive" serological methods turned out to be an understatement. The HHV-6 story was just begining and one could almost say that when HHV-6 finally found its disease, it was the most catastrophic multisystemic pandemic in history.

In the May 9 issue, I wrote an editorial note about something that foreshadowed the *Native*'s rocky relationship with the gay community: "One of our writers showed me a letter he'd received from a friend suggesting that he was bored with the *Native*'s AZT stories. Enough already, the writer implied. This is precisely the kind of attitude the *Native* has had to struggle with since the beginning of the epidemic. Some readers complained when we suggested that there was an epidemic under way seven years ago. Once we won on that point, we were faced with disgruntled readers who felt that our skepticism about the government's claims to have found the cause of the epidemic were out of line. The idea that gay people would trust government scientists working for the current administration is one that historians will ponder for decades to come. It probably will take a mind like Hannah Arendt's to sort through the reasons that so many gay people chose to believe so many lies. If one is a student of the Holocaust, however, one can find many instances in which people collaborated in their own demise. What we need are community leaders who can inspire people to question every statement that government scientists utter about the cause and treatment of so-called 'AIDS.' "

In the May 16 "Chronic Fatigue Report," Neenyah Ostrom interviewed Dr. Paul Cheney: "I recently asked him to describe the neurological symptoms displayed by his 200 CFS patients. Cheney told me that 90% of his patients exhibit 'soft' neurological symptoms, which he defined as symptoms in which the physician is 'struck more by the description than by the exam.' " Ostrom reported, "Hard neurological dysfunction affected 5-10% of his patients." And she noted, "Hard neurological symptoms include seizures, encephalitis, loss of muscular coordination, and weakness on one side of the body."

The amazing thing about Cheney's work, was that it always seemed to be a direct challenge to the "chronic fatigue syndrome is not AIDS" paradigm that was quickly becoming the epidemiological law of the land. But Cheney never played the role—at least not directly or loudly—of the boy in "The Emperor's New Clothes." The neurological symptoms in chronic fatigue syndrome, which Cheney thought were caused by "the elevated levels of gamma interferon, an immune system regulator" should have been a red flag about the connection between AIDS and chronic fatigue syndrome but it was just the beginning of the stubborn and catastrophic denial that would engender unimaginable suffering and cost countless lives.

Despite the *Native*'s reporting, the toxic drug AZT, thanks to AIDS activism and the dearth of critical thinking, looked like it had a very bright future. In the May 30 issue Phil Zwickler reported, "The City of New York plans a wider distribution of the highly toxic and controversial drug AZT, or Retrovir, to prisoners who suffer from AIDS. . . ." Zwickler wrote that New York planned "to identify all inmates who qualify for AZT treatment and insure that they receive AZT." Zwickler wrote, "Many AIDS specialists, including noted researcher Dr. Joseph Sonnabend, maintain that 'AZT is incompatible with life,' and that it is a 'poison' whose adverse effects far outweigh evidence that it prolongs the life of some AIDS patients who take it. Others point out that since quality health care in prison is extremely limited, giving AZT to inmates amounts to cruel and unusual punishment.' " Community activist Philip Reed told Zwickler that coercing the inmates "sounds like institutional genocide to me. In their shortsighted rush to find a solution, they have not looked hard enough."

In the same issue, I once again raised questions about HHV-6, suggesting that Gallo was "trying to sell African swine fever virus as a human herpesvirus, when in fact African swine fever virus is *not* a herpesvirus. It's in a class all by itself. I've talked to three scientists who are growing the DNA virus and none of them is willing to bet their lives that it is a herpesvirus."

I also wrote, "In the May 11 issue of the *Miami Herald*, Rosemary Goudreau reported the following: 'A newly discovered highly contagious herpesvirus might play a role in causing several types of cancer and could be a cofactor in wiping out the immune systems of AIDS patients, one of the nation's premier virologists [Robert Gallo] said Tuesday.' She also wrote, 'Since the AIDS virus kills only a small percentage of T-4 cells at a time. Gallo said the new herpesvirus [HHV-6], if proven to be the cofactor, could explain the total annihilation of T-4 cells in AIDS patients. 'The virus kills cells after using them to replicate, he said.' Goudreau quotes Gallo as saying, 'So if a cofactor is involved in the development of AIDS, and I'm not convinced it's absolutely needed . . . then we want to consider this one strongly.' "

This struck me as being backwards and I wrote, "Wait a minute. If this DNA virus explains the 'total annihilation' of T-4 cells, it seems to me that if a cofactor is involved it would be HIV, not 'HHV-6.' I wish Gallo would stop playing name games with viruses. If this virus is not really a herpesvirus, and clinicians try to treat it with anti-herpes medications, the results could be treatment failure or worse. If the DNA virus is African swine fever virus, then pigs could be used for experiments, rather than AIDS patients. And that way controlled experiments could really be controlled."

I also wrote, "From my discussions with scientists at the Department of Agriculture, I've been able to surmise that in all probability, there is an epidemic of chronic African swine fever in pigs in various parts of the country. As part of a cover-up of this epidemic, the department is stopping most of the research on African swine fever. . . . The department is also retiring a swine fever expert named William Hess, who has complained in the past about the way the USDA has handled testing for African swine fever virus. He was reprimanded for taking his ideas to the press. He has also been the primary source of my information about African swine fever virus for the past five years. I assume that he is being retired because he is something of a whistleblower and because of the information he has given the *Native*. If our nation is now in the middle of a swine fever epidemic in people and pigs, one way to deal with it is to fire everyone who tells the truth. I'm an optimist. It won't work."

Well, it kinda did.

In the May 23 issue, I reported on some shocking information I had found in a recently published textbook on African swine fever virus: ". . . it looks as if we were right about the similarities between 'AIDS' itself and African swine fever. Several officials at the U.S. Department of Agriculture ridiculed our assertions that the two diseases are similar in their clinical courses. In 1984, J. J. Callis, Director of the USDA facility at Plum Island, wrote in a memo, 'Swine ill from ASF show very little clinical similarity to AIDS in man.' A book called *African Swine Fever* by Yechiel Becker, published last year by Martinus Nijoff Publishing, presents the following sea change: 'The ability of ASF virus to infect and destroy cells of the reticuloendothelial system leaves a defenseless host that succumbs to an infection which may be described as an *acquired immune deficiency disease* of domestic pigs [italics mine].' After five years of trying to convince the USDA that this was true, at least it's nice to see that the *Native* was right all along. Wouldn't it have been nicer still if pigs instead of people with 'AIDS,' had been used to test the effectiveness of AZT . . . and other toxic antivirals?"

The in-your-face outrageousness of the Callis lie about AIDS and ASF, was a shocking warning to me about just how far the government was willing to go in deceiving the public about the epidemic. It was starting to appear that the government would do or say *anything* to maintain the epidemic's prevailing AIDS paradigm for the epidemic.

In the June 6 issue, John Lauritsen took the *New York Times* to task for its uncritical report on an AZT trial reviewed by the Food and Drug Administration. Gina Kolata had reported, "Drug company researchers say AZT prolongs life for patients." When Lauritsen looked closely at the study, the news story was based on he found no supporting evidence. Lauritsen found all kinds of anomalies in the study, especially in the way that patients who took AZT and those that didn't were compared. Lauritsen was troubled by the fact that patients on AZT still alive 11 months after they had begun treatment was considered some great kind of victory. The FDA study seemed very disingenuous because, as Lauritsen wrote, "According to an AIDS researcher who was involved in the AZT trials, only a handful of the AZT patients are still alive, and even these frequently had to be taken off the drug and/or given reduced doses."

Lauritsen sent out another warning to the gay community: "It's not easy to keep a clear head in the midst of the current 'health crisis.' The performance of the medical establishment and the media has been abysmal. On all sides we are assaulted by contradictory information. An AIDS mythology, a self-perpetuating delusional system, has developed, and irrationality of all kinds is flourishing."

In the June 20 issue, we published the text of a letter that was being sent out by Ira Glasser, the director of the American Civil Liberties Union. It was another of those "with friends like these" moments in the labyrinth of the epidemic. On the surface it seemed "right on": the letter began, "Will it come to this? Will AIDS sufferers be compelled to wear identifying badges like the Jews in Nazi Germany? Everyone knows that during World War II, Jews were made to wear yellow stars of David. What is not as well known is that homosexuals were made to wear pink triangles. Today in America, some have suggested similar methods to identify and stigmatize people with AIDS. There have even been proposals to tattoo people with AIDS. While such proposals have not been taken seriously, hysteria and fear are already producing astounding examples of inhumanity."

One can't argue with such liberal sentiments, but it is in the well-intentioned details of what the ACLU proposed that one can find the devil. All the ACLU's calls for the protection of civil liberties came wrapped in the almost Orwellian notion that the really bad thing about discrimination was that it prevented patients from getting "the education and medical services they need." The ACLU's calls for confidentiality in AIDS testing completely sidestepped the more fundamental issue of the epidemiological violation of human rights implicit in the HIV test and the anti-gay paradigm it maintained.

As soon as the ACLU joined in the charade of calling for "public education," the organization was unknowingly becoming an enabler of the "chronic fatigue syndrome is not AIDS" paradigm, which, by defrauding the gay community of the uninflected facts of the epidemic, turned the ACLU's crocodile tears about civil liberties into cold comfort. Ira Glasser closed his misguided letter with a statement that perfectly captured the unholy alliance that the civil liberties group was making in the name of helping the gay community: "We don't have to give up our freedoms to successfully fight AIDS. The twin goals of sound public health policy and a healthy respect for civil liberties are not incompatible." What Glasser didn't grasp was that everything about the AIDS paradigm violated what I would call the fundamental *epidemiological rights* of the gay community—the right not to be scapegoated for an epidemic by totalitarian, abnormal science as well as the right to epidemiological truth, something every AIDS patient and every member of the gay community was deprived of (along with the CFS sufferers and other victims of HHV-6).

John Lauritsen summed up the state of AIDS epidemiology in the August 1 issue: "Psychological warfare is being waged against gay men in the United States. For the past month or so, the media has been disseminating hostile propaganda, with the message that we will all die, that we must die. The death threats do not issue from the usual bigots—not from Roman Catholic agitators or menopausal beauty queens or fundamentalist TV hustlers or quack psychiatrists or Hasidic zealots. We are not being drummed to death by voodoo witch doctors or anathematized by prurient priests. We are being cursed in the name of science, and the imprecations directed against us have the imprimatur of the Public Health Service. The prognosis of doom is emanating from that peculiar form of medical survey research known as 'epidemiology.' "

Lauritsen was horrified by the paradigm that was forming, the one that held that all HIV-positives would die. He quoted from an article by Michael Specter that was published in *The Washington Post* on June 3: "The AIDS virus [sic] will almost certainly kill everyone it infects unless effective drugs are developed to treat it, federal researchers have predicted for the first time."

Lauritsen was alarmed that epidemiology-based research would condemn the HIV-positives to be treated with AZT and indeed, Specter confirmed it, reporting, "Public health service officials . . . hope the new study will encourage those at highest risk to be tested so that they will seek medical attention if needed. . . . Many physicians are prescribing AZT for their patients who are infected but have not developed AIDS, although the drug has not yet been proven effective for those patients. Public health officials say that this study is likely to encourage other doctors to prescribe it to patients infected with HIV."

Lauritsen argued that the study Specter reported on did not support the draconian conclusion that was being echoed in the mainstream press. The study of patients in San Francisco, which was published in *Science*, just didn't seem right in the context of what was known then about the mortality of AIDS patients. Lauritsen argued, "A basic principle of analysis is that data must make sense. This may seem too obvious to mention, but novice analysts often are slaves to the numbers they see in front of them, and will concoct bizarre explanations rather than come to grips with contradictions in the data. In actual practice, when data don't make sense, it is almost always because they are wrong." Lauritsen noted that it didn't make sense that at the time in New York City only 1% of HIV positive individuals were coming down with AIDS and, according to the questionable study, 25% of positives in San Francisco were developing AIDS. He asserted, "If HIV is the sole cause of AIDS, it is not possible for both sets of data to be correct."

Lauritsen was sensitive to the way terror of the epidemic was being used to manipulate the gay community. It was daring of him at the time to even say, "I sometimes think that too much attention and sympathy have been given to those who are sick and dying, and not enough to those of us who have healthy minds and healthy bodies. We, after all, are also targets of psychological warfare. We also are increasingly being portrayed as sources of pollution, as threats to the 'innocent' heterosexual population. . . . Our survival depends on not accepting the role of victim. If people direct death wishes at us, we should direct death wishes right back again at them. No one should be allowed to attack us with impunity. At the same time, we need to retain a sense of cool, an appropriate balance of self-preservation, anger, and a sense of humor. Aside from the fact that our lives are at stake, current events are pretty ridiculous, aren't they?"

Michael Dukakis was running for president against Ronald Reagan that autumn, so I was concerned about the person who might become his Secretary of Health and Human Services if he prevailed. In an editorial titled "An Open Letter to Mathilde Krim," I wrote, "There has been a rumor around for some time that you want to become Secretary of Health and Human Services under President Dukakis. In fact, a few weeks ago, a source in the White House told me that he thought it was your obvious objective. I've had many arguments about your motives over the last few years. When I first met you, I found you to be intelligent and charming and witty. Over the last seven years you have come to be celebrated as a great humanitarian. I may be the only person in the world to stand up and say this: I don't trust you or your organization. Nonetheless, I would like to make the following suggestion to you: Let's stop the fraud of HIV once and for all. Your organization has turned out not to be an independent critical force in the epidemic, but rather the handmaiden of the government's lying. Now amfAR has been able to extend its web of lies into Senator Edward Kennedy's office by sharing your Director of Programs and Special Projects, Terry Beirn, with Kennedy's staff, in the capacity of Legislative Aide. I assume that Beirn is there to keep Kennedy from asking the hard critical questions about the real cause of AIDS and Chronic Fatigue and Immune Dysfunction Syndrome [CFIDS]. I believe that Beirn did everything he could to discourage research into the link between AIDS and African swine fever virus. . . . Let's face it, Mathilde, science and life are full of surprises. Who would have thought that after all the pronouncements about HIV, and all the testing, and all the research, and all the conferences, and all the celebrations of the discoverers, that it would turn out that HIV is not the cause of AIDS? While it is a tragedy for the human race, it is kind of a reminder to scientists that they should always keep an open mind and know that experiments—not powerful individuals like Gallo and Myron Essex—are what determine the truth in science. The cost of the HIV mistake and the African swine fever virus cover-up is the Chronic Fatigue Immune Dysfunction Syndrome epidemic. Now that scientists have spent years lying about the cause of AIDS, they are being forced to lie about the cause of Chronic Fatigue Immune Dysfunction."

In the October 31 issue, Neenyah Ostrom wrote a piece about a man in Boston whose plight captured the craziness of the emerging "chronic fatigue syndrome is not AIDS" paradigm. Steven Rose told her, "I've been sick for ten years with what I think is chronic fatigue syndrome, and if I do have AIDS—which I don't think I do—I want the quality of my life to improve *now*. I've spent my entire adult life ill and basically unable to function. I'm one of those 'loose cannons' who never really bought HIV, who never trusted AZT, and who got into this mess by insisting that I be treated for CEBV [Chronic Epstein-Barr Virus Syndrome]. I wound up in a maze of bureaucracy and sheer terror so bizarre that I wouldn't know how to make the movie without Alfred Hitchcock."

Ostrom reported, "Rose was diagnosed with 'AIDS dementia' at Massachusetts General Hospital in Boston. For a time, he participated in the National Institutes of Health Protocol 005 under the direction of Dr. Martin Hirsch of Harvard University, an 'AIDS dementia' study in which participants were given AZT."

Ostrom noted, "Rose doesn't think he has 'AIDS dementia'; he has been ill for ten years with what he believes to be chronic fatigue syndrome (CFS). The symptoms of 'AIDS dementia' are virtually identical to the neurological symptoms seen in CFS patients: forgetfulness, short-term memory loss, difficulty concentrating, impaired judgment, and mood changes (March 1988 *Psychology Today*.) Rose believes that he has been misdiagnosed because physicians are unwilling to admit that CFS exists."

Ostrom also reported, "In the spring of 1987, Rose collapsed while visiting friends in Rhode Island, after a period of time during which he had been working long hours in a stressful job. His friends rushed him to a hospital where he remained for four days." He told Ostrom, "As a gay man I knew the first thing they were going to say was 'HIV.' I didn't think that HIV was the problem, and I didn't want to get stuck in the HIV ghetto, with all my other problems being ignored."

Ostrom reported that Rose was positive for HIV as well as Hepatitis B and that he had high titers to CMV and EBV, telltale signs of chronic fatigue syndrome. He told Ostrom, "Trying to get treatment for chronic fatigue is infuriating and futile. In Boston, Harvard says no to even talking about it—especially with an HIV-positive patient— because they are afraid that you [the *New York Native*] are right . . . I have asked to be tested for HHV-6. . . . But even the 'Gay' clinic won't touch it."

Rose recounted to Ostrom that, eventually, he was told by his psychiatrist that he was not displaying signs of "AIDS dementia," and that he never had it, but, "as a gay man it was the most convenient label for the medical establishment to put on him."

Rose told Ostrom, "If I have AIDS I should be a star patient—a survivor of ten years! In fact, I would go so far to say that I was misdiagnosed—hustled into the HIV-AZT machine—and am perhaps the biggest walking, talking threat to [major AIDS researcher] Marty Hirsh and his cronies around. I never got as sick as they had obviously planned on, and I think I irritate them by being alive at this point."

Rose had found his way into the opposite world created by the bogus totalitarian science that was the foundation of the epidemic. His case was a scientific anomaly that might have awakened the scientific community to the error of their ways, had we been living in a world of normal science.

In the November 14 issue, we published Neenyah Ostrom's report on a CFS symposium that was held in Rhode Island and was attended by more than 300 physicians, scientists, and journalists.

Ostrom reported that pioneering chronic fatigue syndrome researcher, Dr. Anthony Kamoroff of Harvard, told the audience, "Fever is a common symptom; five to ten percent of Komaroff's patients have daily fever, and 40 to 90 percent experience recurrent fever. Twenty percent of his patients experience severe night sweats, and Komaroff emphasized that there is a new finding that physicians should note. In contrast to the fever findings, a number of patients have low body temperatures. A body temperature of less than 98.6 was found in 13 percent, less than 97 degrees in 16 percent, and less than 96 degrees in seven percent" of his patients.

The pathological findings in CFS patients were all over the place, which was one of the reasons that the confusing epidemic would remain hidden in plain sight. It played all too easily into the hands of a medical establishment that seemed determined to sweep the complicated "AIDSish" epidemic under the rug of psychoneurosis.

Ostrom reported that, according to Komaroff, "Like the temperature data, white blood cell counts are both above and below the normal range. Twenty percent of patients have elevated, and twenty percent have decreased, white blood cell counts. In addition, 36 to 41% of Kamaroff's CIDS patients have extremely low sedimentation rates (a test which shows the presence of viral infection) of less than 5; the normal sedimentation rate is around 25. This is a result that is found in people with sickle cell anemia, and led Kamaroff to raise the possibility that a red blood cell membrane abnormality exists in people with CIDS."

Ostrom also wrote that, according to Komaroff, there is often liver pathology in CIDS and "Twenty-five percent of patients have elevated liver enzymes, and develop a non-A, non-B hepatitis at some point in their illness."

Ostrom also reported that there were striking neurological symptoms in Kamaroff's patients: "Disorientation is seen in 15 to 20 percent; each of the following symptoms was reported by approximately five percent of Komaroff's patients: primary seizure, acute profound ataxia (failure of muscular coordination), localized weakness, and transient blindness. Sensitivity to light, blurred or double vision, forgetfulness, distractibility, and peresthesia (an abnormal sensation, such as burning or prickling) also are reported."

That the government refused to acknowledge what was going on, became more and more unbelievable. Government scientists were flatly refusing to legitimize or accept the research findings that were pointing to a picture of an AIDS-like, or AIDS-intertwined, or AIDS-related epidemic in a non-gay population.

In a November 28 article, Ostrom took up the question of how common the syndrome was. She reported, "A number of researchers have expressed concern that the epidemic of CIDS is reaching worldwide proportions, and may dwarf that of 'AIDS.' " Dr. Paul Cheney, the pioneering researcher had written in a CFS journal, "CFS [CIDS] . . . now appears to be . . . epidemic, and generalized across national boundaries. . . . An apparent rise in cases probably from the 1970s in this country and overseas suggests a pandemic." He also wrote, "Despite the increasing weight of evidence that this syndrome is a real disease with measurable immunology, serologic, and neuro-logic abnormalities, many institutions and prominent physicians continue to scoff at this problem and the patients who have it. . . . Quite apart from the professional divisions over this syndrome, this could be a very serious and widespread health problem."

1989: A Strategy Emerges

In the January 2 issue of *New York Native,* in an article titled "Murmurs of the Heart," Neenyah Ostrom discussed some of the more serious pathologies associated with chronic fatigue syndrome: "Spontaneous abortions, heart murmurs and arrhythmias, chest pain, thrush—all of these symptoms of chronic fatigue syndrome (CFS) that appeared in early descriptions of the illness, but have received little emphasis or have faded entirely from the recent literature. All are symptoms that are not included in the Centers for Disease Control 'working case' definition of the disease."

She reported on a study of 189 CFS patients conducted by Dr. Anthony Kamoroff which found that 'atypical pneumonia' developed in five percent of the patients, and that 34 percent exhibited a chronic cough."

She also reported, "In a recent telephone interview, [Dr. Paul] Cheney said that thrush was 'reasonably common' among his CFS patients." Also according to Ostrom, "Chest pain, several types of arrhythmias (a variation in the normal rhythm of the heart beat), heart murmurs and tachycardia (an abnormally rapid beating of the heart) occur in Cheney's CFS patients. He has seen a few patients with 'focal myocarditis,' an inflammation of a section of heart muscle. Mitral valve prolapse is not infrequent in 10-20 percent of his patients. This is a type of heart murmur caused by the prolapse (displacement or partial collapse) of the mitral valve on the left side of the heart."

In the same issue, John Lauritsen brought our readers up to date on the dark progress of AZT and its acolytes: "It's now more than a year since the *New York Native* published my exposé on the Phase III AZT trials which were the basis of the drug's hasty approval by the Food and Drug Administration (FDA). In that article . . . I demonstrated that the FDA-conducted trials of AZT were not merely sloppy, but fraudulent. In the meantime, a lot of water has gone under the bridge. On the one hand, Burroughs Wellcome, the manufacturer of AZT (now known as Retrovir) has launched a worldwide propaganda juggernaut, with great success: the majority of physicians treating AIDS now prescribe and even proselytize for AZT, and thousands of gay men (including those with AIDS, with ARC, and merely with antibodies to HIV) are being dosed with the drug. On the other hand, there is now a groundswell of opposition to AZT."

Lauritsen wrote about a conference that was held at Columbia

University to discuss the state of AIDS treatments. At the panel on AZT, a prominent AIDS activist who had been an "important opponent of AZT" did a complete about face and played down the frightening toxicity of the drug. But AIDS doctor Joseph Sonnabend told the audience "that the toxicities of AZT should not be dismissed lightly." He pointed out, "Never before has a drug as toxic as AZT been prescribed for long term use. The long-term effects of AZT, the cumulative toxicities, are unknown. Sonnabend emphasized the ethical responsibilities of the physician to be sure that there was a sound scientific basis for the benefits of the drug, considering that its toxicities were firmly established."

When Lauritsen tried to ask a question from the audience, Laura Pinsky, the moderator, "screamed that there would be 'no discussion from the floor.' The panel was over." (It was the kind of discourse that characterized the whole epidemic.)

When Lauritsen attempted to question one of the speakers on the panel, a gay doctor named Ron Grossman who had defended AZT turned his back on Lauritsen and when Lauritsen returned to his seat he was approached by a security guard who said he had been asked to "escort" Lauritsen from the building. Lauritsen wrote, "I don't like being silenced, and I don't like having security guards called on me because someone is afraid of my presence: that I might say something out of place or write an article for the *New York Native*. I don't like showcase conferences devoted to creating delusions so fragile that they would be shattered by free and open discussion. This is totalitarianism."

The game the government was about to play for three decades became clearer in a report titled "The Straus Strategy Emerges," by Neenyah Ostrom that we ran on January 23. She wrote about research published by Stephen Straus (Anthony Fauci's CFS puppet at NIAID) and several colleagues that had appeared in the December 29, 1988, *New England Journal of Medicine*. She began her piece with the money quote from the researchers: "Our findings are reminiscent of data showing that psychological factors contribute to one's vulnerability to delayed recovery from acute infections and are in accord with recent findings that a history of affective disorders is frequent among patients with chronic fatigue syndrome."

The researchers showed the government's cards when they asserted, "Although we could not identify a reliable laboratory marker of disease severity, we did find an association between the results of psychological tests and patients' sense of well-being. Significant improvement in levels of anger, depression, and other mood states correlated with overall clinical improvement. These results indicate that affect plays an important part in the perception of illness severity in the chronic fatigue syndrome." Thus did the "CFS is not AIDS" paradigm begin morphing into what would turn out to be three decades of treacherous psychological jabberwocky.

Ostrom noticed the anomalies in the study: "Straus's continued assertions that CIDS 'represents a psychoneurotic condition' and that 'a history of affective disorders is frequent among patients with chronic fatigue syndrome' are rather inexplicable, particularly in light of some of the results that he and his colleagues report. Study participants had 'higher geometric mean titers of antibodies to cytomegalovirus than age-and-sex-matched controls'; three patients displayed antinuclear antibodies (indicative of possible autoimmune disease) and one exhibited a 'low-positive tier of rheumatoid factor' (indicative of possible rheumatoid arthritis). Ten of the 63 blood samples from study patients showed elevated levels of circulating immune complexes (compared to one of 27 from controls); ten of 73 patient serum samples showed elevated levels of the immune system modulator interferon; and levels of an interferon-induced enzyme, 'reflecting the activation of some immune pathways,' were 'higher in patients than in controls' in this study."

Not only *didn't* the data cry out "AIDS" or "AIDS-like" to the researchers, but they wouldn't even admit that what they were seeing was a real disease. Ostrom wrote, "Indeed, Straus appears to have an adversarial relationship with those very people whose illness he is trying to elucidate and ameliorate. He has written that, 'It is difficult and at times unpleasant to address the demands of such [CIDS] patients or to test hypotheses as to the etiology of their woes.' " Ostrom asserted, "Straus demonstrates a healthy disrespect for the information provided by CIDS patients. . . . The language of this report is contemptuous, incorporating such comments as, 'we could not confirm the relentless clinical deterioration reported by some pa-tients.' "

Ostrom captured the disconnect between the science of chronic fatigue syndrome that was going on inside and outside the govern-ment: "Straus and his co-workers are correct in stating that there is currently no 'reliable laboratory marker of disease severity.' [But] while it may indeed be difficult to correlate abnormal laboratory findings with subjective reports of health and well-being, other investigators have experienced no difficulties identifying a myriad of serious clinical abnormalities in CIDS patients, very few of which were identified by Straus et al."

Ostrom reported, "A partial list of such laboratory findings includes: lowered populations of natural killer cells; perturbations in T4/T8 lymphocyte ratios; elevated levels of the immune system modulator interleukin-2, development of brain lesions; elevated liver enzymes, elevated immunoglobulin G, presence of autoantibodies; and decreased cell-mediated immunity." (In other words, like AIDS patients, they were an immunological mess.)

Ostrom pointed out, "In stressing the psychological components of CIDS (which every disease certainly possesses), Straus and colleagues ignore the well-established fact that numerous viruses infect the central nervous system, thereby causing perturbations in mood, cognition, memory, and a host of neurological symptoms."

Ostrom reminded our readers that a "virus which has been isolated from people with CIDS and considered as a possible causative agent, is human herpesvirus-6 (HHV-6 or Human B-Lymphotropic Virus, HBLV)." She also noted that, in a different research project, "Dr. Howard Z. Streicher and collaborators (a group that included Straus) report finding antibodies to HHV-6 in 70 percent of CIDS patients."

The political problem with HHV-6, of course, was that HHV-6 was also found in AIDS patients. That made the virus much too much of an epidemiological hot potato. It threatened the comfort zone of both the AIDS and CFS paradigms which were being maintained by the government's very peculiar "science."

One of the great tragedies of the balkanization of one unified epidemic into a biomedical state of apartheid with a political firewall of bias between so-called "AIDS" and "chronic fatigue syndrome," was that any real scientific progress in one arbitrarily separated part of the epidemic could not benefit its sister epidemic(s). In the February 6 issue of *New York Native* I wrote a piece that tried to capture the tragedy of that epidemiological balkanization: "In 1987, three researchers from the Department of Internal Medicine at Shirnrakuen Hospital in Niigita, Japan, along with one researcher from Pittsburgh, Pennsylvania, published a paper which may have inadvertently resolved the chronic fatigue syndrome/AIDS epidemic, without any of the authors fully realizing what they had accomplished. The paper was published in a journal called *Natural Immunity and Cell Growth Regulation* (1987;6(3):116-28). Anyone who thinks that our crooked, incompetent scientific establishment at the National Institutes of Health has completely screwed up our understanding of the CFIDS/AIDS epidemic should track down this study. The paper reports on 23 patients who were suffering from symptoms that we in American would suspect are part of the Chronic Fatigue Immune Dysfunction and Acquired Immune Deficiency epidemics. The patients had remittent fever and uncomfortable fatigue which had persisted for more than six months. Because the symptoms the patients experienced reminded the physicians of AIDS, the researchers performed tests to determine the status of the patients' immune systems. What they consistently found in the patients was that their natural killer cell activity was lower than that of the general population. They decided that the finding was a definite laboratory abnormality and they immediately sought to correct it." The researchers gave the patients, whom they labeled Low Natural Killer Syndrome (LNKS) patients, 'an immunopotentiator called lentinan, a glucon extracted from the Japanese mushroom *Lentinus edodes*' otherwise known as shiitake mushrooms. According to the researchers, the 'LNKS patients responded well to the administration.' The lentinan was 'administered every other day. Or twice a week intravenously by drip infusion for one hour or injected intramuscularly.' Initially the natural killer cell activity decreased even further, but after continuous administration of the lentinan for six months, the activity returned to the normal range. The researchers also reported 'the return of a feeling of well-being and a disappearance of fever was seen after 2-4 weeks of treatment.' " The researchers noticed that when treatment was discontinued, the symptoms returned.

I also noted, "It seems that the Japanese are way ahead of us in understanding the chronic fatigue syndrome and immune dysfunction (CFIDS) epidemic. Researchers here are still debating whether it exists in reality, or only in the patient's mind. These Japanese researchers may have performed a great service by framing the diagnosis of the disease around an immunological test in combination with several clinical symptoms in a relatively straightforward manner. Indeed, they assert boldly that 'the syndrome is readily detectable by NK assays, and may be treatable with lentinan.' What is the cause of LNKS? The researchers suggest that 'one possibility is that the patients were infected with some unknown virus.' The researchers report that the 23 patients generally have normal T4/T8 ratios, but in some cases they noted a low T4/T8 ratio. When I looked at the T4/T8 ratios of the 23 patients, I noticed that most of the patients had ratios on the low side of normal. Indeed, three or four of the patients had ratios that would have American physicians immediately diagnosing 'ARC' [AIDS Related Complex]."

I also pointed out, "It's my understanding that most AIDS patients have lower NK activity than seen in the general population. It seems reasonable to suspect that in addition to whatever else they're suffering from, they have LNKS, which may be caused by the same agent that is causing LNKS in Japan."

Once again—and it would happen over and over—epidemiologically speaking, AIDS and CFS were two ships passing in the night. Had they been seen then in 1989 as one connected but variable epidemic manifesting a spectrum of illness, both AIDS patients and CFS patients might have had their lives saved or improved by lentinan and the research community would have had a better understanding of the role of NK cells in what was really a pandemic threatening everyone, not just the unpopular risk groups. But once again, tragically, it was not to be.

The chronic fatigue syndrome patients were outraged by the ridiculous Straus research that had been published the previous December. On April 3 we published "The Patients Revolt," an article by Neenyah Ostrom. She reported, "A blistering attack upon 'CFS expert' Dr. Stephen Straus at the National Institute of Allergy and Infectious Disease (NIAID), the National Institute of Health (NIH), and its director, Dr. Anthony Fauci, is delivered in the January/February issue of *The CFIDS Chronicle* [a patient advocate publication]. An editorial and two articles detail the inadequacies and meanspiritedness that characterize Straus and the NIH's lame efforts to address Chronic Fatigue and Immune Dysfunction Syndrome. . . . The charges leveled at Straus and the NIH appear to lay the groundwork for a class action suit on behalf of people with CIDS."

Unfortunately, such a suit never materialized.

Ostrom also reported that the editor of *The CFIDS Chronicle* recommended pressuring "Congress to remove Stephen Straus from his position as 'CFS expert' at NIAID. The two editors wrote, 'Rather than being intrigued and challenged by the complexities of CFIDS, Dr.

Stephen Straus seems to be bothered and disgruntled with its patients and determined to characterize it as a psychological disease. . . . We do not know whether Dr. Straus's failure to illuminate the real nature of this illness is attributable to misguided methods or motives (or both). But we do know that the results of his campaign to 'psychologize' CFIDS are enormously damaging to those who have the disease. . . . Patients are viewed as being morally deficient and somehow responsible for their own illness (as has been the case with AIDS.)' "

The irony of chronic fatigue syndrome patients comparing themselves to AIDS patients would become exponential throughout the next three decades.

The *Native* used the Freedom of Information Act to request all documents concerning chronic fatigue syndrome from the Centers for Disease Control and, as a result, on May 18, we published most of the text of a letter sent to Surgeon General C. Everett Koop by a physician who had been diagnosed as having Chronic Epstein-Barr Syndrome (CEBV), as chronic fatigue syndrome was originally known. The physician wrote, "This letter concerns chronic mononucleosis and the possibility that the contagious but unidentified-as-yet virus causing it is also the trigger for full blown AIDS. I *personally* know many (about 40) health care workers who have contracted CEBV since 1981, all of whom were personally healthy, and all of whom worked with AIDS or lymphoma patients, usually through working in intensive care units, direct patient care, or as oncology nurses or as ear-nose-throat doctors at the time they became ill. I am writing about a highly contagious, rapidly spreading new epidemic in America now occurring that is a more serious threat to our society than AIDS."

The suggestion in the letter that people working with AIDS patients were getting CFS underlines the epidemiological message of this book. But of course it was an epidemiological epiphany that nobody really wanted to seriously think about for the next three decades.

The doctor wrote that he was "a middle-aged board certified physician [who] had the misfortune of contracting 'Chronic Epstein-Barr virus reactivation syndrome' . . . four years ago. I had a productive, satisfying medical practice, prior to that time and had been in excellent health, but awoke with a severe sore throat and flu-like illness one day and have been totally disabled since, solely due to 'CEBV.' There are many thousands of other patients totally disabled by this disease, almost all of whom have caught it since 1980. Like AIDS, the rate of new cases seems to be accelerating."

The physician also speculated, "The cause is a very contagious virus spread like the common cold." He also noted, "The immune system damage and other abnormalities produced by this virus resemble in some ways those found in AIDS patients. The reason that this is a more serious threat to our society than AIDS is that it is spread by much more casual contact, is much more highly contagious, and rapidly spreading. Rather than killing the victims, it renders them permanently disabled. Many are on Social Security Disability. The dollar cost to our society of CEBV is already comparable to that of AIDS and may soon exceed it."

The physician warned, "The CEBV epidemic could have a disastrous effect on our armed services, much more dangerous than AIDS, due to its ability to *rapidly spread like the common cold*. Since it can spread as quickly as it recently did in Lake Tahoe, where over 500 people contracted it within several months, it can quickly disable entire bases, as well as leave a large number of personnel permanently disabled at great expense." (Hello, Gulf War Syndrome.)

In the letter, the physician listed all the immune abnormalities then associated with the disease and named several possible viral causes, including HBLV (or HHV-6) and even African swine fever virus. He also warned Koop, "There is reason to believe that the same virus that causes CEBV causes many lymphomas."

The physician presented his own game plan: "There should be the appointment of an accomplished *senior* investigator, who has a track record of success in identifying new pathogens, to spend *full time* heading the NIH's CEBV program. Another accomplished investigator should be appointed to head the CDC's CEBV program. Power similar to that of a general in war time should be given to these senior officials. This would help ensure full and rapid cooperation of competing labs and scientists working on these problems."

Well, that didn't happen.

Other documents we received, from our F.O.I.A. request, captured the exasperating games the CDC was going to play with chronic fatigue syndrome for three decades. On May 22 we published an exchange of letters between the CDC's Gary Holmes, and Dan Peterson, one of the two Incline Village (Lake Tahoe) physicians who discovered and characterized the CFS epidemic in their area. Peterson wrote to Holmes, "I would like to update you on the current conditions at Lake Tahoe. We now have nine patients who have developed B-cell lymphoma from the original study group that had evidence of reactivated herpes diseases in the form of elevated early antigens for Epstein-Barr virus and tissue culture positivity for human herpesvirus-6." Holmes wrote back to Peterson, "The case histories of the patients you presented in the letter are quite interesting. However, I believe most of the researchers in the field agree that CFS is a diagnosis of exclusion, and that the identification of other diseases, such as lymphomas that occurred in your patients, or of MRI abnormalities that are suggestive of multiple sclerosis (MS), moves such patients out of the CFS category. CFS is little more than a collection of symptoms at the present time, and it remains highly likely that many patients' CFS symptoms are actually caused by occult lymphoma, multiple sclerosis, or any of multiple other chronic diseases that may not be diagnosed in the initial evaluation. Continued grouping of patients who have such definitive diagnoses as lymphoma or MS under the title of CFS may artificially imply that such patients have a single cause for their varied illnesses."

That is how the game of CFS Three-Card Monte would be played for the next three decades. One couldn't even begin to point out that CFS was part of the AIDS epidemic if serious complications of CFS were constantly and disingenuously used to undermine the very diagnosis of CFS itself. By CDC fiat, no CFS patient would ever be seen as suffering from AIDS-like secondary infections and of serious CFS complications. Neenyah Ostrom summed up the diagnosis problem: "The circular reasoning applied in this instance appears to be a classic case of throwing the baby out with the bathwater: if the diagnosis of CIDS is one of exclusion, and the subsequent development of a known illness (such as cancer) removes the patient from the subset of people with CIDS, not only will the possibly progressive nature of the illness never be investigated—a specific diagnosis will not be developed. At least not by the CDC."

The transformation of the gay community into the HIV Pink Triangle Community made a great deal of progress that summer. According to the *New York Post*, the New York City Health Commissioner, Stephen Joseph was planning to call for the collection of the names of everyone who tested positive for HIV. The Health Department denied that any plan was in the works and released the complete text of Joseph's speech that was given at the annual AIDS conference in Montreal. The ideas in the speech were chilling enough. In his speech Joseph said, "It is only a matter of time before reliable published studies demonstrate the effectiveness of treatment for the asymptomatic HIV-infected person, or for preventing infection in an exposed person, or for reducing infectiousness of the person with HIV infection. These changes in our capacity to prevent and treat infection will usher in a new era in which policies will shift towards a disease control approach to HIV infection along the lines of classic tuberculosis practices. Medically confidential counseling and testing both become more aggressive and routine in high prevalence areas of all clinical settings. Within a confidential public health framework, reporting of seropositives, follow-up to assure adequate treatment, and more aggressive contact tracing will become standard public health application for controlling HIV infection and illness."

Anyone who knew what a massive political fraud the HIV paradigm was felt like they were staring into the depths of hell when they realized what Joseph was calling for. To politically force AIDS into a TB paradigm was frightening because TB patients could be arrested and quarantined in prisonlike conditions if they did not cooperate and take the state's prescribed treatment. It was one thing for the AIDS establishment to say what it thought the cause of AIDS was and what treatments might be the most helpful. This was different. The state was about to turn its theories or mistakes, depending on your viewpoint, into law. It was diabolically brilliant.

The AIDS activists were worse than useless in the face of the approaching totalitarian darkness that Joseph's agenda represented. Their opposite world activism was driving the growth of this horrifying AIDS empire. A couple of letters we published, in the June 19 issue, captured the degree to which the AIDS activist community was turning the gay community upside down. At the beginning of June there had been a ceremony in Manhattan's Sheridan Square to celebrate Gay/Lesbian Pride and History Month. The ceremony, which was attended by the mayor of New York, was disrupted by ACT UP. Jim Puzio of San Francisco wrote, "Instead of a ceremony honoring the Lesbian/Gay community for the achievements over the past twenty-five years, I saw a demonstration by ACT UP in which the mayor and other speakers were shouted down. Instead of feeling proud, I was embarrassed. In my view, and that of others I spoke with that day, what was ruined was one of the accomplishments of the Lesbian/Gay

Rights movement—to be recognized by the city government and have our voices heard. I wouldn't blame the mayor if he never did another thing for the Gay/Lesbian community. . . . At the ceremony I was handed a flyer urging me to join another demonstration at the Pride Rally. If ACT UP is going to screw up that also, I think I'll stay home."

Another reader, Walter J. Phillips, wrote, "ACT UP's action at the unveiling of Stonewall Place in commemoration of the Stonewall riots was a disgrace. AIDS, while very tragic, has only been with us a few years, while gay oppression has existed for hundreds of years. When the highest elected official chooses to speak about that oppression in a manner to give hope and courage to all gay people, the chanting of ACT UP and prevention of those who wanted to hear from doing so was misguided to say the least. While both AIDS activism and gay activism are necessary and desirable, actions must be constructive and beneficial to the gay community."

We published another letter in that issue on a different matter that provided more evidence that not everyone in the gay community was being bamboozled by ACT UP's deceptive activism. Don C. Olson had dared to point out at an ACT UP meeting "that they have lost their focus since challenging the HIV theory is a major issue in fighting AIDS. Well, all hell broke loose, since my sentiments were too controversial for them, because they are fixated on the HIV/AZT/let's find a vaccine rot. To put it mildly, I caused a big stir. Several members accused me of disrupting the meeting. I said I thought this was ACT UP (had I come to the wrong place?). They tried to sweep me under the carpet by suggesting I talk with their HIV-Treatment Committee. Well, I did approach their HIV-Treatment Committee and (pathetically) all they wanted to discuss was HIV treatment. . . . I am furious with S.F. ACT UP'S dangerously narrow perspective, and with N.Y. ACT UP's boycott of the *Native*. They are sadly misinformed, because they choose to ignore (and in this case, resist) new findings published by such responsible papers as the *New York Native.* . . . And in so doing, ACT UP members perpetuate right-wing style censorship at the cost of continued suffering of their gay brothers and sisters. (I guess ACT UP has moved so far to the Left, it has become part of the New Right.)"

In the June 26 issue, Neenyah Ostrom covered CFS research pioneer Dr. Paul Cheney's testimony to Congress concerning the CFS epidemic. Cheney told Congress that CFIDS might have a relationship with the AIDS epidemic. He also said that one informal "survey of patients in CFIDS groups from 35 states shows an exponential rise in cases produced each year since the 1970s. This curious temporal and case production relationship with the AIDS epidemic has prompted some researchers to project CFIDS as an AIDS epiphenomenon. Indeed, the new human herpesvirus HHV-6 may be about the most important cofactor shared by both AIDS and CFIDS."

A report by John Hammond, in the July 3 issue, once again captured the cockamamie nature of AIDS activism. At a breakfast meeting which took place in New York City's Gracie Mansion with Mayor Koch in June, a prominent group of "health care professionals and other experts involved with the City's response to the 'AIDS' crisis firmly rejected Health Commissioner Steven Joseph's suggestions, originally aired in a speech before the Fifth International AIDS Conference on June 4, to give serious consideration to the possible use of coercive measures in responding to HIV infection."

Hammond reported, "These measures included adopting 'confidential' (as opposed to the current 'anonymous') procedures for recording HIV-antibody tests, mandatory reporting of positive test results, and involuntary contact tracing and notification for all persons who tested positive for HIV antibodies. Most health care advocates and professionals agree that such methods are unlikely to be productive in this epidemic, where many people at risk fear discrimination, and there is evidence that where such measures have been tried, as in the state of South Carolina, they have discouraged many from seeking diagnosis or treatment."

In the same issue, we ran a fascinating interview with Dennis King conducted by Neenyah Ostrom. King is the author of *Lyndon LaRouche and the New American Fascism*. The interview is a reminder of how easily the CDC's biased epidemiology could be used for all kinds of vicious right-wing agendas. King told Ostrom, "You've got to understand that, two years ago there was an enormous scare in our society about AIDS. Now it's like everything else—it hits television, and people become somewhat inured to it. People are still worried about it, but the hysteria two years ago was a media event. And LaRouche knew this was a golden opportunity for some demagoguery. So he called his followers together, and gave them a slogan—and if you ask me for a *classic* slogan of demagoguery, I couldn't come up with a better one. LaRouche said, 'Spread panic, not AIDS.' I think that the panic was there, especially with people believing that AIDS was going to spread very rapidly into the heterosexual community, which it didn't, but at the time people were worried that it would do so. The hysteria was out there in the land and LaRouche had no difficulty getting 700,000 people to sign a petition to put that referendum [Proposition 64] on the ballot. What happened next is even more interesting. The people who were opposed to Proposition 64 formed a committee called Stop LaRouche. They publicized all over the state the fact that Lyndon LaRouche, the dangerous extremist, was behind this measure. And that anti-LaRouche agitation apparently had very little effect on people's voting patterns. People didn't care. They were worried about AIDS, and they couldn't care less that it was a Nazi behind it. When the election took place, the *New York Times* reported—without giving any statistics— that the referendum had been overwhelmingly defeated and that it was a great victory over LaRouche. Bullshit. LaRouche got over two million people in California to vote in favor of quarantining a minority. It was a great victory for him and for the forces of neofascism in America. For the first time, they had inserted into the public mind the idea of rounding up a minority, and inserted it in such a way that people could feel it was legitimate, by disguising it as a public health measure. And LaRouche learned how to do that from *Mein Kampf*. If you look at what was going on in our society at that time, the AMA [American Medical Association] poll [that found that 50 percent of Americans thought it was okay to deprive people with AIDS of their civil liberties] was really minor compared to the enormous violence that was erupting against gays all over the United States. And the violence is continuing today. And that is something that is not being looked at closely enough by people who should be concerned, like the government, civil liberties groups, Jews—who after all, are the next target, because it's skinheads doing it. They may beat up on gays now, and they may beat up on blacks, but the ultimate target is the Jews. It always is in these situations. . . . LaRouche has praised skinhead attacks on gays, openly, and he has called the skinheads the 'vanguard of the nationalist revolution.' "

In the July 24 issue of the *Native*, Ostrom raised the question of whether Gilda Radner, the *Saturday Night Live* comedienne, was a victim of chronic fatigue syndrome: "Gilda Radner died on May 20 at the age of 42, following a long illness that culminated in ovarian cancer. But three years before her death, and, approximately a year before the diagnosis of cancer was made, Radner was told she had . . . 'Epstein-Barr virus' disease" as chronic fatigue syndrome was then known.

Ostrom asked, "Did Radner develop ovarian cancer from the chronic immune dysfunction caused by 'chronic fatigue syndrome?' " Radner had written a book about her illness called *It's Always Something* and her description of a cold that would never go away, as well as the fog that filled her brain, low-grade fevers, and a panoply of other symptoms matched the pattern that was seen in CFS patients all over the country. Radner, like many or most of the patients in those days, was told she was suffering from depression or neurosis. Ostrom sarcastically wrote, "In October 1987, Radner's 'neurosis' resulted in abnormal liver function tests. That same month, the ovarian malignancy was discovered—almost a year-and-a-half, by her chronology, after Radner experienced the cold that wouldn't go away." Ostrom concluded her piece by asking, "How long will it be before serious research on this debilitating illness is begun by U.S. health authorities? How many lives must be destroyed—and perhaps lost— while desperate patients go from doctor to doctor, like Radner did, being told that their symptoms are psychological?"

In that same issue, Ostrom noted that *The Washington Post's* Michael Specter had reported on a rather troubling alliance that was forming between the government and the AIDS activists. In the July 9 report, on a meeting in D.C., Specter wrote that federal officials "had gathered here today with community activists from around the country to discuss ways to dramatically speed the distribution of experimental new AIDS drugs." While it was a huge victory for the activists, it opened up AIDS to all kinds of scientific confusion in which adverse side effects might not be recognized in an orderly way. Drugs would not be tested as rigorously as they had been in the past. That was what was considered progress in the new opposite world the AIDS activists were helping to create. Specter never wrote more truthful words in his entire career than these: "Fauci and some other AIDS researchers have begun to sound almost as if they were shadow spokesman for groups like ACT UP." (A vice versa version of that statement is also painfully true.)

Meanwhile, in the same issue, we reported on the tragic story of a drug that AIDS patients had been experimenting with in the process of doing their own clinical trials on themselves. John Hammond reported that a number of deaths had been caused by "Compound Q or GLQ233, a chemical extract made from the root of a particular variety of Chinese cucumber." Hammond wrote, "Compound Q, long used for other medical purposes in China, became a matter of near-hysteria among some 'AIDS' patients when, on April 13, Dr. Michael McGrath of the University of California in San Francisco (UCSF) published his finding that, in a test tube, the drug completely destroys human macrophages previously infected with so-called Human Immunodeficiency Virus (HIV) and, apparently, only those cells. The drug is also highly toxic and this spring two people with 'AIDS' nearly died after eating homemade cucumber root preparations."

Hammond reported that, "In the case of Compound Q, Project Inform, a San Francisco-based 'AIDS' information organization headed by Martin Delaney, decided to sponsor its own trials of the drug, in an effort to make the drug more readily available to patients willing to participate in trials and in order to speed up the overall approval process. Instead of minimal test dosages, the Project Inform trials combined Phase I and Phase II testing and began with larger, therapeutic dosages of Compound Q, tested on 42 patients. One patient in the Project Inform trial committed suicide and a second lapsed into a coma and choked to death on his own vomit. In New York, a third patient who was not part of the Project Inform trial but who had obtained the drug on his own, died after taking his second dose under a doctor's supervision." Such stories were emblematic of the tragic desperation that characterized those dark times.

In the July 31 issue, Neenyah Ostrom reported on a fascinating experiment conducted by Japanese researchers that may have re-flected the best understanding to date of chronic fatigue syndrome. As previously noted, the Japanese had, instead of using the goofy moniker of chronic fatigue syndrome, focused on a measurable biomedical marker and called the malady "Low Natural Killer Cell Syndrome." Ostrom reported, "A group of researchers led by Tadao Aoki at Shinrakuen Hospital (Niigata, Japan), together with Dr. Ronald B. Herberman at the Pittsburgh Cancer Institute, defined 'Low Natural Killer Cell Syndrome' (LNKS) in 1986 (before the U.S. Centers for Disease Control even published its case definition of chronic fatigue syndrome). They defined LNKS as 'a newly proposed category of immune disorders, being characteristically diagnosed by lowered NK cell activity . . . in association with general clinical symptoms of remittent fever and uncomfortable fatigue, persisting without explanation for more than six months.' " The scientists speculated that the cause might be "a new, unknown virus or an unknown substrain of known viruses."

Once again, the tragedy was that AIDS also was obviously a form of Low Natural Killer Cell Syndrome. The overlapping nature of these politically separated epidemics was met by radio silence. It is especially tragic because the Japanese researchers also discovered that intravenous lentinan (derived from shiitake mushrooms) could turn the condition around. The games the CDC was playing with CFS prevented it from being recognized as treatable LNKS. The American government's scientific establishment seemed determined not to let doctors or the public see CFS as an epidemic of immune compromised people, let alone AIDS. God only knows how many people would still be alive today if the American government had adopted an LNKS paradigm for both CFS and AIDS, and attempted to control the real epidemic with lentinan.

In that same issue, Ostrom reported that Fauci's department (NIAID) was "sponsoring a new clinical trial to evaluate the safety of AZT in pregnant women who are infected with the human immunodeficiency virus (HIV)." Ostrom noted, "The stated aim of the study is to determine 'whether AZT given during pregnancy can prevent the transmission of HIV from mothers to their newborn babies.' " She pointed out, "At a time when most responsible physicians urge pregnant women not to take so much as an aspirin if it can be avoided, how can NIAID possibly justify giving a drug as toxic as AZT to pregnant women? Poisoning black babies after birth apparently isn't good enough. . . . The government will now poison black babies *in utero*."

Ostrom also noted, "According to the *New York Times*, 52 percent of women and 76 percent of children with 'AIDS' are black even though blacks compose only 12% of the general population." ("Black Doctors Urge Study of Factors in Risk of AIDS," by Felicia R. Lee, *N.Y. Times,* July 21, 1989.)

One of the more horrific passages from the Fauci press release about the AZT experiment on pregnant black women stated, "During labor, they will again receive intravenous AZT until the infant is born."

As I studied the issues of the *Native,* in the process of writing this book, it was surprising how much of a treasure trove the letters to the editor will be for future historians of the epidemic. We published two that were stunning in the August 7 issue. A German writer named

Kawi Schneider had just become familiar with the *Native* and wrote, "Unfortunately, I got to know your brilliant newspaper criticism of 'AIDS' not before yesterday. In a future article, I will describe your brilliant resistance against AIDSzism. My grandfather was in a social democrat anti-Nazi resistance group. When I see how victims of the 'AIDS' misdiagnosis are killed today with poisons (like AZT) that even the healthiest people wouldn't have a chance to survive long-term, I more and more come to believe that we have a U.S.-based reincarnation of Nazism in only slightly different disguise. And again, good and naïve people are being abused to do the holocaust job. Again, resistance is too weak. Again, dissenters are being ridiculed. Again, there is a Führer cultism (if you doubt this, just join the next Gallo-worship AIDS conference). . . . AIDSzism is not just a concealed renaissance of Nazism, but it is also a strategy to annihilate modern medicine and modern science."

In the same issue, we published a letter from Stephen F. Temmer, another person who was not hoodwinked by what was happening in the gay community. Temmer wrote, "In arranging for the meaningful distribution of my charitable funds, I was struck by the incongruity of Gay Men's Health Crisis donating funds to ACT UP, a strictly political, and I dare say, counterproductive group. I wrote a letter to Richard Dunne, GMHC's Executive Director and he responded with a thoughtful, two-page letter indicating that GMHC as a tax exempt organization is permitted by law to funnel up to 5 percent of its contributed income to organizations it supports, even though such organizations may not themselves be eligible for tax-free status, as is the case with ACT UP. I feel very strongly that organizations involved with the care of people suffering with AIDS should stay strictly out of the political arena and leave such work to those not primarily involved with the community's suffering. I am sure it cuts deeply into their ability to raise the needed funds for their urgent work and on that basis alone it should preclude their supporting controversial groups." While Temmer may have made a very practical point, the money flowing into ACT UP from GMHC was evidence that ACT UP was getting its political claws (the ones that were also basically bolstering the government's epidemiological agenda) into every aspect of gay life.

In the same issue of the *Native*, I wrote an editorial expressing my concern about a new toxic drug, DDI, that had been touted by the *New York Times*: "Gina Kolata's *New York Times* report on Friday, July 28, on DDI will be hailed by many with the same enthusiasm that greeted the early stories on AZT. While doctors' phones will start ringing off the hook, let us at least note that the DDI story acknowledges what a toxic disaster its predecessor AZT was. Without qualification, that is something to celebrate. At the same time, the ghost of AZT (and we do hope it will become a ghost) should offer a cautionary tale about DDI and other chemotherapies that may take center stage. The people who have voted to boycott the *Native* are the same ones who have demonstrated to lower the cost of AZT or to make the drug available for free."

I also pointed out, "The *Native*, thanks to the persistent analytical work of John Lauritsen, has been a lone voice in calling attention to the dangers of AZT. Even though we faced a boycott by ACT UP, we continued to tell the truth about AZT. Two months ago, when NYC Health Commissioner Stephen Joseph announced his plans for contact tracing and the adoption of a tuberculosis model for the containment of 'AIDS,' I asked an official in the Health Department if that meant that people would be contacted and encouraged to take the appropriate treatment. The official said yes, and that he assured me that the treatment would be AZT because it has been shown to extend life.' "

Kolata had written in the *Times*, "In a study of 26 patients, being reported in the journal *Science*, the 23 patients who received the highest doses of the drug [DDI] showed increases in their immune system cells, decreases in AIDS viral proteins in their blood, as well as weight gain. Three even had a reversal of their dementia."

But she also reported that Sam Broder, the Director of the National Cancer Institute, "warned that the drug could still have dangerous side effects. At very high doses, higher than those in the new study, researchers have found that DDI may damage the pancreas or aggravate nerve problems in the hands and feet that can lead to difficulty in coordination."

I was very alarmed by what seemed to be the appalling logic that was emerging and wrote in the editorial, "One issue of concern to us is that DDI is being compared with AZT to make sure it is a better treatment. What a standard to hold DDI up to! The fact that DDI is less toxic than AZT should not come as much of a surprise to anyone familiar with the awesome toxicity of AZT."

The chronic fatigue syndrome patients, who were in essence sitting in the front of the government's fraudulent epidemiological AIDS/CFS bus, while lucky not be turned into clueless toxic dumps like the folks in the back of the bus, had their own problems to contend with. In the same issue of the paper, Neenyah Ostrom wrote a piece about their inability to obtain insurance benefits: "The Centers for Disease Control's definition of chronic fatigue syndrome . . . as an illness with a 'diagnosis of exclusion' has created a myriad of difficulties for physicians, patients and health insurance providers. One of the potentially most explosive—and expensive, in terms of the public health, as well as money—is that insurance companies have begun to deny reimbursement to some, if not all, expenses related to [chronic fatigue syndrome]."

John Lauritsen was back on the AZT case, in the August 21 issue of the *Native*. He noted, "The AIDS industry has not given up on the drug. There is apparently a huge stockpile of AZT, and billions of dollars of sales depend upon a continued, and expanding, market for the commodity."

Lauritsen was outraged that Tony Fauci's National Institutes of Allergy and Infectious Diseases (NIAID), which had sponsored the AZT study (that was terminated early), had issued a press release, "in which Anthony Fauci called the results 'exciting' and urged that AZT be given to all of the estimated 100,000 to 200,000 Americans who, like the study participants, are somewhat sick and have HIV antibodies. Another study is currently in progress, testing the effects of AZT on *perfectly healthy* people who have HIV antibodies. If equally 'exciting' results can be obtained from this study, the AZT market may explode to as many as 1,500,000 hapless Americans."

Lauritsen noted, "After a little investigation I found out that the much touted AZT study has not been published in any form, very little is known about it, and much of what was said in the media reports is not true. . . . NIAID's press release was reprehensible in many ways." Lauritsen argued, "With regard to AIDS coverage, the media are exquisitely cognizant of an 'elite consensus'—the consensus of the AIDS establishment. The consensus consists of a paradigm, an elaborate mythological system, which though its tenets sometimes change, is so well internalized by most AIDS writers that they could recite the basic catechism in their sleep: AIDS is a deadly new disease, which is invariably fatal, which is caused by HIV. Intravenous drug users got AIDS by 'sharing needles.' Gay men got AIDS by being 'promiscuous.' AZT 'extends life' and is the 'best hope.' All or nearly all of those who are 'infected with HIV' (have HIV antibodies) will get AIDS. Africa is a continent ravaged by the AIDS epidemic, with millions of people sick and dying. And so on. Facts that don't fit into the official paradigm transmute into unfacts [and go down the] memory hole. The propaganda model suggests that mainstream AIDS coverage might best be understood as collusion between the media and parts of the Medical Industrial Complex. It suggests that we always keep in mind the economic underpinnings of the epidemic."

The gay community's unfortunate cooperation with its own epidemiological persecution and humiliation was starkly captured in a piece written by James D'Eramo, in the September 11 issue. He wrote, "Joining with long standing federal recommendations and the recent barrage of media coverage urging widespread HIV antibody testing and AZT use, Gay Men's Health Crisis (GMHC)—in a break from its cautious stance on these issues—has endorsed what can be seen as essentially the government's often stated and most recently emphasized position. In his swan song press conference at GMHC office, on Tuesday, August 15, Executive Director Richard Dunne (he has since resigned) read a statement saying, 'There are compelling reasons to get tested and to know your HIV status.' Dunne cited a New York State law that protects confidentiality, and the availability of 'drugs which can prolong life by slowing the development of AIDS' as the 'compelling reasons' for testing. In GMHC's concurrent testing campaign print ad, 'Think about it,' only AZT is mentioned by name as one of the drugs that can slow AIDS onset."

D'Eramo noted, "Over the past months, there has been a highly orchestrated national campaign urging that all those at risk of being exposed to AIDS be tested for the presence of antibodies. The federal government health agencies, and local public health officials, including New York City's Health Commissioner, Stephen Joseph, have recommended that the names of persons who test positive be reported—and kept on a 'confidential' list—and that their contacts be tracked down, tested and listed as well."

D'Eramo also noted, "For years now, many psychosocial professionals, physicians, scientists, civil rights activists, and AIDS organizations—including GMHC—have pointed out that the HIV antibody test could actually cause an individual more harm than good." Perhaps most disturbingly, D'Eramo reported that when Dunne was asked at the press conference if GMHC had received a grant from Burroughs Wellcome, "Dunne said he did not know the exact amount, but it was used exclusively for client services rather than for salaries or operating expenses. For some, the fact that the not-for-profit organization first accepted money from the AZT manufacturer, then later recommended extensive use of the drug, has created an impression of impropriety."

GMHC was making the trains run on time.

Before I discuss another piece by Neenyah Ostrom that was in the same issue, I must quote the uncanny first two paragraphs of Randy Shilts's *And the Band Played On*. They inadvertently reveal how epidemiologically intertwined AIDS and CFS were at ground zero:

> Tall sails scraped the deep purple night as rockets burst, flared, and flourished red, white, and blue over the stoic Statue of Liberty. The whole world was watching, it seemed; the whole world was there. Ships from fifty-five nations had poured sailors into Manhattan to join the throngs, counted in the millions, who watched the greatest pyrotechnic extravaganza ever mounted, all for America's two-hundredth birthday party. Deep into the morning, bars all over the city were crammed with sailors. New York City had hosted the greatest party ever known, everybody agreed later. The guests had come from all over the world.
>
> This was the part the epidemiologists would later note, when they stayed up late at night and the conversation drifted toward where it all started and when. They would remember that glorious night in New York Harbor, all those sailors, and recall: From all over the world they came to New York.

It's a shame the attention of those same AIDS epidemiologists didn't also focus on the September 11 issue of the *Native*, in which the article by Neenyah Ostrom, on a gay man with chronic fatigue syndrome, began, "The long downward spiral of illness for Rich Jones began on the night of the Fourth of July, 1976. It was the culmination of the nation's Bicentennial celebration and 24-year-old Jones was excited by New York City's festivities. 'That Fourth had a Disney-like quality,' he remembers. He and a friend sat on the dunes, watching the fireworks over the Hudson River; they built a small fire, and stayed up all night, drinking and talking and celebrating the country's two-hundredth birthday. Walking home in the early morning, Jones suddenly felt quite ill. 'Something is wrong,' he said to his friend. 'I feel very sick.' 'Of course you feel sick,' Jones's friend replied. 'You've just stayed up drinking all night.' 'No, that isn't it.' Jones insisted. As it turns out, it wasn't. That night was the turning point in Jones's life, a change in his health that was, he now says, 'very, very, very dramatic.' Jones has chronic fatigue syndrome. That morning, a 13-year odyssey through illness began."

The rest of Ostrom's piece describes Jones's struggle and the details of his illness were not all that different from the other patients that Ostrom would interview and profile during her eight years of reporting on CFS. But it was an amazing coincidence in the opening of his story that one gay man's chronic fatigue syndrome also began at the precise moment in time that epidemiologists suspected AIDS had begun in America. It was an epidemiological Tweedledum-Tweedledee moment for AIDS and chronic fatigue syndrome, a moment that supported the notion that the two epidemics had been politically separated at birth.

As I have argued, if the real epidemic had not been sexually, socially and racially divided epidemiologically into a kind of medical apartheid, the tragedy of genocidal AZT might have been averted. At the very least, the Cassandras who were concerned about AZT might have been listened to with more respect. Ostrom interviewed one of those Cassandras, in the September 18 issue of the *Native*.

Dr. Bernard Bihari, a member of the Community Research Initiative, was a pioneer of research into relatively nontoxic treatments for AIDS like naltrexone and lentinan. While he believed that AZT could help patients who had AIDS dementia, he was concerned about giving AIDS patients AZT in the early phase of their illness. In addition to HIV resistance, he was concerned about "some long-term cumulative toxicity. . . . We may be doing more harm than good. . . ." He was mindful of the fact that one could not project long term effects of AZT on studies that had only lasted a year. Interestingly, he noted that the early studies "showed reduction in opportunistic infections." In the next two decades many critics would argue that the anti-AIDS drugs were not helping because they targeted HIV, but because they had broad spectrum effects against the dozens of infections that AIDS patients (and CFS patients, by the way) suffered from.

In the October 2 issue, Ostrom wrote a piece titled "The

Andromeda Strain" which looked at the reasonableness of the possibility that chronic fatigue syndrome was actually caused by African swine fever virus, a virus (we later learned) that may have been circulating undetected in America's pigs with immune system problems for a number of years—under the disingenuous diagnosis of "swine mystery disease" and eventually porcine respiratory and reproductive syndrome (PRRS). Ostrom noted, "One of the more compelling arguments for a multifactorial explanation of chronic fatigue syndrome . . . is the improbability of a single pathogen being capable of causing the wide range and variable severity of symptoms seen in the illness. Numerous systems of the body are affected by CFS—the immune, nervous, muscular, circulatory, and endocrine systems all experience some form of dysfunction. Even the reproductive system may be affected."

Ostrom asserted, "The multifactoral explanation of the cause of [chronic fatigue syndrome] may, in fact, be simply a reflection of how little is known about the illness. But the central question remains: is it possible that a pathogen exists that could cause the wide-ranging symptoms and variance in severity that is seen in [chronic fatigue syndrome]?"

Ostrom looked at the possibility that African swine fever virus, which had been proposed by Jane Teas as the cause of AIDS, was also the cause of chronic fatigue syndrome. She pointed out that African swine fever "is an example of an illness that affects many biological systems: the immune, circulatory, nervous, gastric, reproductive, and pulmonary systems are affected in both acute and chronic forms of the disease." While she didn't say it in the piece, behind the scenes we were wondering if AIDS was acute ASFV and chronic fatigue syndrome was a chronic form of the disease.

Ostrom wrote, "It may seem silly to look at a pig illness when searching for a paradigm for CFS, but human and porcine immune systems are extremely similar. In fact, pigs are a major repository for human influenza viruses, and passage from humans to pigs and back to humans accounts for the wide variety of strains of influenza from year to year." She also noted, "African swine fever, despite the identification of its causative agent and several well-defined clinical courses, remains a truly mysterious illness. It renders the infected animals' immune system unable to respond by mechanisms that are still unexplained; it can cause fever, arthritis, nervous, and immune system dysfunction, skin lesions, pneumonia, susceptibility to bacterial infections, miscarriage, and can lead to death through cardiac insufficiency or coma. Or it can evolve in an infected population into a chronic form, in which relapsing fever, malaise, and other symptoms continue over months or years."

In her summary of the ASF-CFS hypothesis, she noted, "There is no data linking ASF virus to [chronic fatigue syndrome]. But as a model system, ASF would seem to be appropriate. As a model system, it proves that a single agent could in fact be responsible for the myriad of symptoms exhibited by people with [chronic fatigue syndrome]."

Neenyah Ostrom summed up where we were, in terms of the relationship between AIDS and chronic fatigue syndrome, in the November 27 issue. She wrote, "The continuing furor over the Centers for Disease Control's name, 'chronic fatigue syndrome,' for what has been called, at various times, chronic mononucleosis, Chronic Epstein-Barr virus Syndrome, post-viral syndrome and a host of other names, is a good example of how a name can be chosen to dramatize, trivialize, or clinically describe an illness. The number of patient support groups that refuse to use the name chronic fatigue syndrome—many of them substitute 'Chronic Fatigue and Immune Dysfunction Syndrome'— also is testament to the power of a name."

Ostrom also noted that a disturbing game was also being played with AIDS at the same time: "There is an ongoing movement to have Acquired Immune Dysfunction Syndrome, 'AIDS,' renamed 'HIV disease.'" She suggested that the two diseases of immune dysfunction "be renamed to recognize what is probably the most serious infectious agent they have in common: Human B-lymphotropic Virus (HBLV, also called human herpesvirus-6 (HHV-6)." She pointed out, "HBLV [HHV-6] infection may constitute the initial attack on the immune system, weakening it and allowing opportunistic—usually bacterial— infections and transformed (cancer-causing) cells to grow out of control. . . . HBLV is clearly more lethal to immune system cells than is HIV and infects a large number of types of cells—T- and B-cells, macrophages, monocytes, megakaryocytic, glioblastoma cells (cells of the nervous system), and muscle cells. In fact Gallo and co-workers claim that the primary target for HBLV is T-cells, the cell depleted in 'AIDS' and other immunodeficiencies."

In that same issue, we published the first roundtable discussion by the editors of the *Native* about issues related to the epidemic. The topic was a survey then being conducted among gay men in Minnesota about their sexual activities and drug use. Some AIDS activists in Minnesota were concerned that it was a continuation of the state's "unrelenting prying into the sex lives of gay men." John Hammond started the discussion off saying, "I recall a friend, about 15 years ago, blowing up and saying, I'm sick of being studied, and sick of being counted, and sick of being analyzed, and why doesn't someone start treating me like a human being? And this whole thing has the potential for resulting in the kind of sex surveys that Magnus Hirshfield ran in the twenties and thirties [in Germany] that got people to answer exactly such questions, and then after 1934, Hitler used those surveys to round people up."

In the course of the roundtable, I said, "There's the deeper question of sex and the epidemic of chronic fatigue syndrome. They're not interviewing Gene Wilder, for instance—we believe that Gilda Radner died of [chronic fatigue syndrome]. Should Gene Wilder be questioned about his sexual behavior with Gilda Radner? Or, for example, Cher has chronic fatigue syndrome—should all her sexual partners be tracked down? No, it wouldn't happen. Because the paradigm involves basically scapegoating gay people for an epidemic that's widespread, and still mired in fraud and bad science."

In the December 18 issue, John Lauritsen wrote one of his most alarming reports on AZT: "AZT causes cancer in animals. This finding was divulged by Burroughs Wellcome, manufacturer of AZT . . . in an advisory sent on December 5 to thousands of physicians who treat AIDS patients. Widespread consternation ensued. Confused and contradictory statements were issued to the press by physicians, Public Health Service officials and 'AIDS activists.' " Lauritsen reported that the conclusion of the study which involved "60 male and female rats and mice" was pretty clear: "No tumors were found in any of the control rodents," but a significant percentage of the rodents given AZT developed cancer.

If the AIDS establishment was shaken by the finding, they kept it to themselves because, according to Lauritsen, "Immediately promoters of AZT rushed in to downplay the significance of the findings. In an Associated Press story, Dr. James Mason, Assistant Secretary of the Department of Health and Human Services, said the results 'do not establish that the drug has a carcinogenic effect in humans.' Along the same lines, Burroughs Wellcome stated in its letter that 'results from rodent carcinogenicity studies are of limited predictive value for humans.' These are strange things to say. If rodent carcinogenicity studies have little 'predictive value for humans,' why do them in the first place? If rodent studies are meaningless, why are they a standard part of the toxicity screening of new drugs?"

Lauritsen was troubled by some of the the reactions to the study: "In responding to news about the rodent carcinogenicity studies, a number of AZT apologists sounded a peculiar theme: The risks of AZT must be weighed against its benefits." Lauritsen noted that one activist had been quoted in the mainstream press as saying he was more afraid of AIDS than cancer. Lauritsen wasn't having any of it and wrote, "There is a large and growing body of information on the risks of AZT. In addition to the risk of cancer, AZT . . . destroys the bone marrow and causes severe anemia; it damages the kidneys, liver, and nerves; it causes severe muscular pain and atrophy (wasting away). What then are the 'benefits' of AZT that could offset such terrible toxicities? I have maintained, and continue to maintain, that there is no scientifically credible evidence that AZT has benefits of any kind."

In that same issue, we took up the subject of AZT in another editorial roundtable titled "Concentration Camp without Walls." I opened the discussion saying, "Let's discuss whether prescribing AZT is a form of genocide or not."

Ron Gans was critical of the gay groups that were cooperating with the authorities who were promoting AZT: "It's an amazing circumstance when you have groups that are born in opposition to the established order deferring to the established order. The whole purpose of groups like Lambda, all the gay groups, all of them, is an opposition to challenging the established order. . . . It boggles the mind. The only conclusion I can draw from this is that people have always trusted the government, deep down they always have." I made this remark about ACT UP's involvement with AZT: "Why would anybody want to take a drug that has been approved because people sat in somebody's office and wouldn't leave until they okayed that drug? That's what scares me about AZT." John Hammond suggested, "Maybe there's an area . . . that the entire movement has never thought through and that nobody has talked about very much and that is, is there a way to get leverage and apply pressure and get results in which you're not making research decisions or forcing research decisions in a way that warps them and makes the scientific evidence illegitimate?" Neenyah Ostrom pointed out, "People keep saying, 'I'm not a scientist. I can't question HIV or Robert Gallo's work.' But those very same people feel capable of saying, 'Give me this drug, make this drug available now.' They didn't say 'I'm not a scientist, I can't decide whether this drug is good for me or not.' "

I said, "You know it's interesting, the risk that some activist organizations are taking with AZT. The odds really are against them, the odds are that all these people that are pushing [and taking] AZT are going to be dead. . . . You'd have to be hoping for a miracle for that not to happen. . . . People with AIDS—many of whom probably haven't had much access to medical care—are now in the medical system for the rest of their lives. They're in a concentration camp without walls. . . . If only they were giving AZT to dogs we'd have the animal rights groups on our side. They wouldn't allow it."

Notes

Introduction

p. 11.   "woodenheadedness." Barbara Tuchman, *The March of Folly* (New York: Random House Publishing Group, 1984) p. 7.

p. 11.   "self-deception." Ibid.

p. 11.   "fixed belief." Ibid.

p. 11.   "evidence to the contrary." Ibid.

p. 11.   "a policy . . . hindsight." Ibid., p. 5.

p. 11.   "a feasible . . . available." Ibid.

p. 11.   "that the policy . . . individual ruler." Ibid.

p. 12.   "Poison Kitchen." Ron Rosenbaum, *Explaining Hitler: The Search for the Origins of His Evil* (New York: Random House, 1998) p. 37.

p. 12.   "nemesis." Ibid.

p. 12.   "the persistent . . . in his side." Ibid.

p. 12.   "The Munich Post . . . toward Berlin." Ibid.

p. 12.   "a dozen years." Ibid., p. 38.

p. 13.   "they knew . . . his skin." Ibid.

p. 13.   "It was . . . life miserable." Ibid., p. 40.

p. 13.   "the Hitler Party." Ibid.

p. 13.   "Their repeated . . . criminal pathology." Ibid.

p. 13.   "men such as . . . its limits." Ibid., p.42.

p. 13.   "even glimpsed . . . in the Third Reich." Ibid.

p. 13.   "as a homicidal . . . political party." Ibid., p. 52.

p. 13.   "the shocking . . . horrifically true." Ibid., p. 53.

p. 13.   "According to Rosenbaum . . . bitter end." Ibid., p. 53

p. 13.   "to restore . . . combat with [Hitler]." Ibid., p. 59.

1981-1984: The Fog of Epidemiology

p. 15.   I had asked Dr. Lawrence Mass, in May of 1981, to look into rumors of a rare form of cancer striking men and in the May 18, 1981, issue of the *New York Native* we ran a story with the headline "Disease Rumor Largely Unfounded." Dr. Mass wrote, "Last week there were rumors that an exotic new disease had hit the gay community in New York. Here are the facts. From the New York City Department of Health, Dr. Steve Phillips explained that the rumors are for the most part unfounded. Each year, approximately 12 to 14 cases of infection with a protozoa-like organism, Pneumocystis carinii, are reported in the New York City area. The organism is not exotic, in fact, it's ubiquitous. But most of us have natural or easily acquired immunity."

p. 20.   Jane Teas has a Ph.D. from Johns Hopkins University.

p. 22.   Arnoux, Emmanuel, JeanMichel Guerin, Rodolphe Malebranche, Robert Elie, A.Claude Laroche, Gerard Pierre et al.; "AIDS and African Swine Fever" ; *The Lancet*, July 9, 1983, p. 110.

1985: Throwing Down the Gauntlet

p. 40.   Ann Giudici Fettner and William A. Check wrote *The Truth About AIDS: Evolution of an Epidemic* (New York: Henry Holt & Co., 1984).

p. 42.   Nick Wade and William Broad wrote *Betrayers of the Truth: Fraud and Deceit in the Halls of Science* (New York: Simon and Schuster, 1983).

p. 68.   "The first . . . all conditions." Hess, William, "African swine fever: a Reassessment"; *Advances in Veterinary Science and Comparative Medicine,* Volume 25, 1981, pages 36-39.

p. 80.   "The purely . . . were doing." Young-Bruehl, Elisabeth, *Hannah Arendt: For Love of the World* (New Haven, Yale University Press, 1977), p. xiv.

1986: A New Virus or a Renamed Old One?

p. 89.   One of the people who accompanied American officials to Haiti in order to help eradicate ASFV by killing the entire the pig population came back with a mysterious chronic illness. I lost touch with her and I don't know if she ever got better.

p. 92.   The misuse of funds at the CDC may be a chronic problem. Hillary Johnson details the misuse of CDC funds in their mishandling of research into chronic fatigue syndrome in her book, *Osler's Web: Inside the Labyrinth of the Chronic Fatigue Syndrome Epidemic* (New York, Crown Publishers Inc., 1996

p. 93.   Hannah Arendt discusses the nature of governmental image-making and propaganda in her essay, "Truth and Politics," in *Between Past and Future: Eight Exercises in Political Thought* (New York, Viking Press, 1961).

p. 98.   We portrayed Robert Gallo on the cover of *New York Native* as Carmen Miranda.

p. 98.   To really get a sense of Gallo's shocking antics and habit of threatening people, read John Crewdson's *Science Fictions: A Scientific Mystery, A Massive Cover-Up and the Dark Legacy of Robert Gallo* (Boston, New York and London: Little Brown and Company, 2002).

p. 102. Statements like those of Dr. Peter Skrabanek inspired me to start doing some serious critical thinking about the political nature of epidemiology. Before long I was thinking of it as the used car salesman area of "science."

p. 104. If the kind of sabotage that seemed to be going on at the CDC had been occurring in any other area of the government, the media would have assigned its best investigative reporters to cover it.

p. 108. "It was an act . . . was Lysenko." Nicholas Wade and William Broad, *Betrayers of the Truth: Fraud and Deceit in the Halls of Science* (New York: Simon and Schuster, 1986), pp. 187-188.

p. 109. " . . . Himmler was not . . . theoreticians as well." Richard Plant, *The Pink Triangle: The Nazi War Against Homosexuals* (New York: Henry Holt and co. and New Republic Books, 1986), pp. 88-91.

1987: An Epic Epidemiological Battle

p. 115. James H. Jones, *Bad Blood : The Tuskegee Syphilis Experiment: A Tragedy of Race and Medicine* (New York, The Free Press, 1982).

p. 116. John Lauritsen's books on AIDS are *Poison by Prescription: The AZT Story* (New York: Asklepios, 1990), *The AIDS War: Profiteering, and Genocide from the Medical Industrial Complex* (New York: Asklepios, 1993) and with Ian Young, *The AIDS Cult: Essays on the Gay Health Crisis* (New York: Pagan Press, 1997).

p. 120. Darrell Yates Rist co-founded the Gay and Lesbian Alliance Against Defamation. He is the author of *Heartlands: A Gay Man's Odyssey Across America* (New York: Dutton, 1992).

p. 128. I was very disappointed that Vidal never really took his usual cold hard look at AIDS and never helped raise the public profile of the epidemic's critics and skeptics.

p. 132. That wasn't my only contact with the White House. During the Bush Sr. administration I reached Bush's personal physician in the White House and talked to him about the chronic fatigue syndrome epidemic. He was polite and seemed interested, but I got nowhere.

1988: The Public Relations of the Epidemic

p. 137. Harvey Bialy is the author of *Oncogenes, Aneuploidy, and AIDS: A Scientific Life & Times of Peter H. Duesberg* (Berkeley: North Atlantic Books, 2004).

p. 143. "vital lie." Daniel Goleman quoting Henrick Ibsen, *Vital Lies, Simple Truths: The Psychology of Self-Deception* (New York: Simon and Schuster, 1985) p. 16.

p. 143. "a family myth . . . comfortable truth." Ibid., p. 16.

p. 143. "We are piloted . . . psychological life." Ibid., p. 241.

p. 144. "acceptable dissent." Ibid., p. 248.

p. 147. The three books we published by Neenyah Ostrom are *What Really Killed Gilda Radner?: Frontline Reports on the Chronic Fatigue Syndrome Epidemic* (New York: That New Magazine, Inc. 1991), *50 Things You Should Know About the Chronic Fatigue Syndrome Epidemic* (New York: That New Magazine, 1990) which was republished as a mass market paperback (New York: St. Martin's Press, 1993), and *America's Biggest Cover-Up: 50 More Things Everyone Should Know About the Chronic Fatigue Syndrome Epidemic And Its Link to AIDS* (New York: That New Magazine, Inc., 1993).

p. 149. My favorite fact about Mathilde Krim comes courtesy of her Wikipedia entry: "Krim then moved to New York and joined the research staff of Cornell University Medical School following her 1958 marriage to Arthur B. Krim—a New York attorney, head of United Artists, founder of Orion Pictures, and advisor to Lyndon Johnson. It was at Krim's NYC home on May 19, 1962 that the famous 45th birthday party for President John F. Kennedy was held, with many famous persons in attendance (Robert Kennedy, Marilyn Monroe, Maria Callas, Jack Benny, Harry Belafonte)."

p. 154. "The ability . . . of domestic pigs." Yechiel Becker, *African Swine Fever* (Boston: Martinus Nijhoff Publishing, 1987) p. IX.

p. 156. Michael Specter eventually became a writer for *The New Yorker* where he continued to enforce the AIDS establishment's dogma. In the March 12, 2007 issue of *The New Yorker* he wrote a piece titled "The Denialists: the dangerous attacks on the consensus about H.I.V. and AIDS."

1989: A Strategy Emerges

p. 162. We'll never know how many people died of heart attacks which were complications of so-called "chronic fatigue syndrome."

p. 163. Laura Pinsky and Paul Harding Davis wrote *The Essential AIDS Fact Book: Newly Revised and Updated* (New York: Pocket, 1996).

p. 163. Ironically, Stephen Straus died of brain cancer on May 14, 2007. The virus HHV-6, which has been linked to CFS and AIDS is also known to be involved in brain cancer. While the CFS patients often portrayed Straus as the central villain in the CFS cover-up, they seemed to be giving a free ride to his boss at NIAID, Anthony Fauci.

p. 167. If medical workers with CFS had formed their own organization to publicize the CFS epidemic, it could have had a huge impact. Unfortunately, most remained in the closet. It is kind of an open secret in the CFS community that many of the people treating or researching CFS themselves have CFS. The whole issue of CFS being transmitted from health care workers to patients (and vice versa) is one of the many taboo subjects in the CFS community.

p. 172.   Paul Cheney eventually opened a clinic devoted to treating chronic fatigue syndrome in North Carolina. Patients have described seeing Cheney as a fairly expensive proposition. On the Cheney Clinic's website there is a relatively benign—almost watered down—description of the disorder: "Chronic Fatigue Syndrome is a disorder of unknown cause characterized by significant functional disability associated with fatigue, pain and neuropsychological complaints."

p. 173.   Dennis King, *Lyndon Larouche and the New American Fascism* (New York: Doubleday, 1989).

p. 176.   Project Inform was started in 1984 by Martin Delaney and Joseph Brewer. Delaney died in 2009. From a National Institute of Allergy and Infectious Diseases press release issued on January 22, 2009: " 'Millions of people are now receiving life-saving antiretroviral medications from a treatment pipeline that Marty Delaney played a key role in opening and expanding,' says NIAID Director Anthony S. Fauci, M.D. 'Without his tireless work and vision, many more people would have perished from HIV/AIDS. He is a formidable activist and a dear friend. It is without hyperbole that I call Marty Delaney a public health hero.' "

p. 182.   "Tall sails . . . to New York." Randy Shilts, *And the Band Played On: Politics, People and the AIDS Epidemic* (New York: St. Martin's Press, 1987) p. 3.

p. 185.   It became clearer throughout the epidemic of AIDS/CFS that one of the most important political aspects of epidemiology is the power to name diseases. It is not a science but rather a social act of demarcation that always has the unrecognized potential to stigmatize while appearing to being doing something utterly objective and humane. Epidemiology has all the public health propaganda tools it needs to create what Noam Chomsky calls "manufactured consensus."